YouthLift

Also by M. J. Saffon

The 15-Minute-a-Day Natural Face Lift

M. J. SAFFON'S

*Youth*Lift

How to Firm Your Neck, Chin, and Shoulders with Minutes-a-Day Exercises

WARNER BOOKS

A Warner Communications Company

A Warner Communications Company

Distributed in the United States by Random House, Inc., and
in Canada by Random House of Canada, Ltd.
Printed in the United States of America
First Printing: October 1981
10 9 8 7 6 5 4 3 2 1
Book design by H. Roberts Design

Library of Congress Cataloging in Publication Data

Saffon, M. J.
    M. J. Saffon's YouthLift.

    Includes index.
    1. Beauty, Personal.   2. Skin—Care and hygiene.
3. Skin—Aging.   4. Face—Care and hygiene.   5. Chin—
Care and hygiene.   6. Neck—Care and hygiene.
7. Shoulder—Care and hygiene.   8. Exercise for women.
I. Title.   II. Title: YouthLift.
RA778.S194 1981   646.7'5   81-4637
ISBN 0-446-51230-3   AACR2

To Jon Jon,
a camp in life,
yet very brave
in the face of death.
We all miss you so.

Preface

A great many people, with good reason, are concerned about cosmetic problems. Such problems can prevent people from getting what they want—a good job, or even a feeling of well-being. People live longer now, and they want to feel and look their best into their fifties and even sixties and beyond. The retirement age is going up, and it all works together—look good, feel good.

You don't have to be beautiful to be attractive; but you must be alert and healthy, and vital. There is an old saying, "usually a person who looks good is in good condition and is actually a pleasanter person." Exercise plays a vital part in any program designed to achieve that goal.

Interestingly, facial exercise is helpful both without a facelift or in conjunction with a facelift. I believe that facial exercise works. It does a great deal to tone the facial and neck muscles, to give the face a look of firm and alert youthful energy, and to help normalize contours.

—Willibald Nagler, M.D.
New York Hospital–Cornell Medical Center

Special Note

The reader is urged to use personal judgment in performing any of the activities and exercises described in this book, and in applying any of the natural beauty treatments. Any adverse reactions, including muscle strain or muscular or physiological adverse reactions, as well as allergies to any fruits or vegetables, should be taken into account. And, those activities or formulas should be avoided. Of course, no miracles from any beauty care—organic, muscular, or otherwise—should be expected or can be guaranteed.

Dear Readers

Since the publication of my book, *The 15-Minute-a-Day Natural Face Lift*, I have received hundreds of letters asking the same question that students and others have asked me over the years. Even Merv Griffin, the charming and handsome television talk-show host, asked this question when I was his guest: What can I do about my neck?

You need not bemoan the seemingly irreversible effects of age on the neck and shoulders. If you feel that your neck and shoulders are not as beautiful as they might be and that the pouchy skin on your lower face announces your age, I can help you.

The exercises, tips, suggestions, and grooming rules presented in this book have all been tested by my students and others—and they work! The skin areas we deal with in this book are the most difficult to restore, but *it can be done*, and thousands of people are doing it. All you have to do is follow the directions given here for a few short minutes several times a week.

In a few weeks, you can be a show-off. You can display your smooth, round, soft shoulders, your glorious, graceful neck, and your smooth, firm jaw—and you'll look and feel years younger.

This step-by-step program shows you how to rejuvenate your skin so that it is vibrant and flawless and attracts admiring stares and approving glances. Throw off your scarf and high collars—you can wear the feminine and flattering low-necked dresses and casual clothes.

The program described in this book includes exercises and specific skin-care rituals, and it also shows you how changing your posture, smile, and eating habits can give your neck, chin, shoulders, mouth, and jaw a new youthful set and a firm delightful contour.

Enjoy life at its fullest, knowing you look your best from any angle. Go where you want, select the clothing you've long wanted to wear, and feel confident at all times. You can start right now. The program is easy, fast, and reliable.

Keep your chin up! And keep your eye on the stars—you'll soon look like one.

M. J. Saffon

Acknowledgment

Through the years, many friends, students, clients, and doctors have urged me to write about my techniques and to describe the exercises for *YouthLift*. I have held back, thinking that perhaps only through personal consultation could the techniques be taught. At the urging of Helen Gurley Brown, however, and with the help of the editorial, production and art departments of Warner Books, *YouthLift* came into being.

I want to thank all the hundreds of people who have attended my lectures and seminars and the many people who have written me and honored me with their trust and who have relied on my advice. I offer my thanks also to the medical advisors and clinical experts who responded with such enthusiasm to *YouthLift*.

Sincerely,

M. J. Saffron

Contents

YouthLift

PART I

What You Should Know About Looking Young Forever

Why Is the YouthLift Needed?

Have you ever noticed that many well-exercised, slim and trim women have wrinkled, sagging, or dull skin on their necks and shoulders and that their mouths and jaws are far older looking than their bodies? This can happen to the most slender and athletic women, as well as to people who have gained weight with age. Why do some parts of the body seem to show age before others?

Some parts of the body show age before others because we give these areas more or harder wear than other areas; because they are less protected, and because skin varies in thickness, strength, and structure. The thinnest skin is on the eyelids, neck, and the backs of the hands—and these are the areas that show age first.

These thin-skinned areas—the eyes, hands, and neck—are in almost constant motion—they flex and bend as you move. As the mouth, eyes, neck, chin, and shoulders are rubbed or moved, the skin over and around these areas also moves. The problem is compounded by the fact that there are very few oil glands in these areas, so the skin dries and flakes in these areas first. Because we need to use these areas all the time, it is inconvenient to keep this skin covered all the time (as you usually do the skin of the torso), these most delicate areas fall victim to cold winds, harsh sunlight, drying air from heaters, and irritating pollution.

Now that you know why these areas are the most prone to age, you can, with the simple program in this book, retard that aging process and restore your skin's elasticity. As you replenish the muscles under the skin to bring back the smooth glow of youth, you will learn special tricks and techniques to protect the skin over these muscles.

The skin does have enemies—but it also has good friends. Be your own best friend, and recognize and combat the causes of aging in your skin. The glow of youth will return faster and more easily than you think.

3

The Skin's Enemies—
And How to Conquer Them

The best way to avoid aging is to combat the aging process. That means you must avoid all the habits and behaviors that can age you. Here are some of the worst age makers, the real enemies of beauty, and some of the ways you can combat those enemies. First, be aware of the negative influences as you work and play in daily life. The exercise program will achieve results—but those results can be multiplied in effect if you learn to protect your skin from its enemies.

Weak Muscle Tone

Gravity, the same force that pulls us downward and keeps us on the earth, constantly pulls downward on our skin. After several decades of this never-ending pull, the skin on the face and body sags slightly, as the muscles under the skin and the tendons that hold the muscles to the bones weaken, or stretch. (It is easy to see this effect when the skin under your chin sags.) Famous beauties rest on slant boards, or do yoga; they spend hours upside down to reverse this process. But such measures are impractical for most of us. And they are not necessary because within your own body you already have gravity fighters you can use.

Muscles act against gravity; without muscles we would not be able to move or walk. Your face is covered with ribbons of muscles and your neck is overlaid with a large, strong, flat muscle. With age, the muscles in the face and neck gradually shrink, and the fat pads that support them thin or vanish, making the skin over the deteriorated muscle fibers and slack tendons seem too large. It is the loss of this firm muscular underpadding, and the loss of skin elasticity, that creates excess skin that sags, pouches, and wrinkles.

Inactivity is an enemy of fitness, beauty, youth, health, and muscle tone in your body—and your face and neck. To look young, your face, neck, shoulders, and body need the strength and grace that only active youthful muscles and strong elastic tendons can supply. The exercises in this book will strengthen your muscles. They were developed and tested for firming the chin and neck, and they "work" little-used muscles in the most beneficial way.

The special miniprograms will work on your specific problems with your muscles; they will activate, flex, strengthen, and plump and tighten just the right muscles to restore your youthful good looks. Because the muscles of the face are interwoven, they are hard to exercise, and because the muscle of the neck is broad and flat, it loses its firmness easily; *but with the right movements that focus on just the muscles that need exercise, done the correct number of times,* the results will be fast—and amazing!

Weather

You protect nearly all the parts of your body with clothing—especially when the wind blows or the temperature drops. But you usually leave your chin and neck uncovered. The use of scarves and mufflers is some help against the drying of the skin, but open collars and short hair often leave the neck exposed.

It is usually easier to remember to bundle up in cold weather than to remember to avoid the deceptively soothing sun. When you are cold, you automatically reach for something to cover and protect your skin, but the warmth and solace of the sun invite you to expose yourself too long. Take, for example, the "V" of skin often exposed by an open collar in the summer. If you compare this portion of your skin to another area of the body that is covered even in summer, you will readily see how clothing effectively protects the skin from weather-aging.

Summer's air conditioners that dry the air and blow drafts on your neck and shoulders, and winter's central heating that dries skin to parchment-paper flakiness, are also enemies of skin beauty. They are man-made weather but they can be as detrimental to your skin as Mother Nature's own weather.

Sun

Don't go out in the noonday sun. The poets were right—and in many tropical climates women never venture from their homes without the protection of a wide-brimmed hat or an umbrella.

Although you are more aware of the sun's rays on a clear day, you are not safe from the destructive rays on a cloudy day. Seventy to 80 percent of the ultraviolet rays with the power to burn can penetrate clouds on an overcast day. Swimmers must be especially aware of the power of the sun; water is no safeguard.

The result of too much sun is prematurely aged skin. Many people believe the Vitamin D from the sun source is important; but vitamins can be derived more safely from a well-balanced diet. Another reason to sunbathe is the youthful look of an evenly tanned skin. It is hard to believe, but true, that today's tan can easily become a tough leathery hide that suffers from weakened elasticity, invites dark patches and scaly gray-colored growths which should be examined carefully by your doctor.

Your skin is not fully protected even if you stay in the shade of a beach umbrella, for the dangerous ultraviolet rays are only partially deflected by the shade. Rays can bounce off any substance and ricochet in all directions.

Beware of the sun, and follow the advice given below.

- Don't sunbathe between eleven in the morning and three in the afternoon—this is when the destructive rays are most intense.
- Don't use a sun reflector—ever!
- Avoid the sun when you are taking any medication—the drugs in combination with the sun can be very harmful.
- S. P. F. (Sun Protection Factor) information must now be included on the packaging of all sun-protection products. The higher the SPF number, the greater the degree of protection provided. Use number 15 or higher for protection for your face; use number 8 or higher on your body.
- Before applying any sunscreen, spray your face and body with mineral water to ensure an adequate moisture level for your skin.
- Wind—even a cool wind—can rapidly evaporate your skin's moisture. Wind can hasten the drying and uncomfortable feeling of sunburn. Dry skin is unprotected skin.

A suntan is not conducive to a beautiful complexion, and it is not even good for you; it can be foolish and even dangerous. Direct rays of the sun age the skin; sometimes the effects are irreversible.

Direct rays of the sun—the kind that you get when lying on a sunny beach—dry much of the moisture and natural oils out of the tissues. The results are very much like speeding up a clock or calendar; your skin can be aged years in just months. Thickening of the outer layer of the skin cells, loss of elasticity, spotty discoloration (often called liver spots), scaly and wart-covered areas on the neck and shoulders or the backs of the hands, and patches of furrowed skin can be some of the effects of the sun on the skin.

The nose is very sensitive, and dilation of the delicate blood capillaries and blood vessels can result from too much sun. Enlarged pores, broken veins, and an angry red color that is sometimes called "drunkard's nose" can come from the sun. Nature never intended the human body to be overexposed to a baking sun.

Dehydration

How much water do you drink? Your skin can be thirsty. Drink, drink, drink—water and more water, at least eight full glasses of water each day. Not only will your skin look fresher, but you'll feel better, all over. The amount of water you drink can make a big difference in how moist, soft, dewy your skin is. If you drink enough water daily, protect your skin from drying winds and hot sun, and exercise to aid the circulation of blood to your growing skin cells, your skin will never look parched and dehydrated.

Dehydration makes your skin dry, and when it is dry it thickens and becomes dull. The top dry cells will seem flaky instead of firm and bouncy. Dry skin doesn't protect your body as well as moist skin. Notice that after splashing water on your face and neck, your skin looks softer and clearer. It seems to absorb some of the precious water—and, in fact, it does. Capture that beauty-making moisture by protecting your skin with creams and moisturizers. You should also moisturize your face and neck as often as possible by misting your skin. (Directions for making your own mist-spray are on p. 21.)

To fight dehydration, you must drink water so that you have plenty of liquids internally while you protect your skin's surface by retarding the evaporation of the liquids from your skin by protecting it from the outside. Water makes you more attractive—and also makes you feel and perform better.

Water has always been considered the best of nature's beauty and health aids. The ancients—priests, physicians, sorcerers, beauties—recognized its value, particularly the special properties of some mineral spring waters. In every culture, great beauties visited mineral springs and spas and bathed in or drank the water. Internally, wa-

7

ter is the great source of strength and life. Externally, it is the great healer, cleanser, and purifier.

Drinking six to eight glasses of water daily, in addition to the water in tea, coffee, and other beverages, will aid in the elimination of wastes and will flush away toxic materials that clog the pores and cause blemishes.

Most people do not think about water and accept it as always available and uniform in quality. Neither assumption is correct. Water can differ in mineral content as well as organic matter, the color varies from crystal to yellow, to gray, to bluish. No human being can live more than a few days without water. Every vital function, and of course the blood itself, requires about five pints of water every day.

Don't worry about water retention—your body will actually retain less water as it utilizes water effectively. It is the spices in foods, the salts, caffeine, tannic acid, and fats that upset your natural water use. Ordinary tap water, the kind that is found in almost every section in this country, is probably one of your most important beauty aids.

Bottled water, once considered a beverage used only by the elite—presidents, athletes, European nobility, and the super-wealthy—is now available in most supermarkets. Before buying any bottled water, carefully read the label. And, as with any other product you eat, drink, or apply to your skin, be sure that the water has a low-sodium content.

There are famous mineral springs and special waters in almost all countries. One of the most famous in the United States is in Mountain Valley, Arkansas. Spring water is different from man-made mineral waters. Natural mineral water is untreated—no gas, colorants, sugars, or flavors have been added, and nothing is removed or changed in an industrial process.

The best mineral waters flow naturally under carefully guarded and hygienic mountain springs that have a valued reputation. Uniform taste, mineral content, clarity, and color, as well as the specific content of the water, are unchanging and reliable. Many health and beauty spas have grown up around natural mineral springs because the therapeutic values of the spring waters attracted visitors.

If you do not drink enough water and do not mist your skin enough you allow your body fluids to evaporate, your skin will become dehydrated. Without these fluids you strain your entire body—and the strain will show almost immediately on your skin. Dry and rough are your enemies; bright, clear, pure water is your best beauty friend.

Stress

Tension, strain, and tightening of the muscles around your shoulders, neck, and head can result in backache or headache. The tightening of those muscles can decrease the flow of blood through these vital areas and weaken your entire body.

Many doctors believe that stress is the source of several severe illnesses, and our modern world is full of stress. Some call it worry, anxiety, or nerves . . . it is all the same. Each person has her own stress makers. You must learn to recognize yours because they are the enemies of your health and beauty.

What can you do? Turn to the breathing exercises on pages 69–76—these breathing exercises will help immediately. (Actually, all the exercises in this book are stress fighters.) Concentrate on each position as it is described, and clear your mind, especially of negative thoughts. You will be fighting stress, and enjoying a beauty bonus of a smooth firm skin as well.

Diet

Since skin constantly renews itself, you can grow smooth, beautiful new skin at any age. The cells take about three weeks to form and come to the surface, and then, after a few days, they flake away. Certain nutrients are required for the creation of the new cells. Your diet will be reflected in your skin in a very short time—just weeks.

Sweets, spices, and salts are not good skin builders; what skin tissue needs are proteins, vitamins, and minerals. Proteins are very important to your skin. They are also important to your hair and nails. Hair, nails, and skin continually renew themselves and are mostly protein. You also need foods that contain roughage to keep your digestive system working well. A smooth-working digestive system prevents reabsorption of bodily wastes and keeps your skin clear and blemish free. A balanced diet of high-protein foods and some roughage will help you achieve the best muscle- and skin-building results.

Poor nutrition is the enemy of beauty and health. Be sure you are getting the kind of nutrition you need. The quality of the food you eat can be more important than the quantity. The freshness of produce is an important factor in vitamin content. Check all the labels on packaged foods and note the amount of protein listed. (If you are in doubt about minimum daily adult requirements for protein, vitamins, and so on, write to the U.S. Food and Drug Administration, Washington, D.C., for this information.)

You

Yes, you can be your skin's worst enemy! If you habitually slump when you sit, have poor posture when you stand or walk, stretch your skin when you wash or apply creams and makeup, these will eventually weaken your skin and the elastic tissue that ensures a tight hold between muscle and skin, and a firm glowing youthful look.

Stand tall to reduce your waist, lift your cheeks and jowls, firm your neck, and even think more clearly. Practice pushing up as if you are aiming to touch the ceiling with your head. As you do, you'll feel your neck lengthen, your shoulders pull back, and your chest rise. You'll look younger and better instantly.

Sit tall. Keep your head up, your shoulders up and back, and don't allow your torso to slump. The muscles that support your body are damaged by slumping, and the muscles of your neck and face suffer as well. Good posture means better breathing, and stronger and healthier lungs bring more life-giving air into your entire system. Vitality and alert responses are a breath away.

Your fingers are a miracle of nature—they can pick up the tiniest objects, yet they are strong and flexible. Don't touch your face with them—don't rest your chin on your hand, don't pick or pull at your chin, face, or ear. (You might do these things without being aware—check with a friend.)

Grimacing and Other Bad Habits

Grimaces, gestures, mannerisms, tics—these habitual facial movements will eventually put wrinkles, creases, and folds in your face.

This is a NO-NO list. Here are some expressions and grimaces that age you immediately. Each time you affect one of these mannerisms, you are forming your face into an age-making position:

- Compressing your lips to form a displeased look
- Sucking at your teeth
- Tensing your mouth so that your lips are drawn inward in a small straight line
- Pursing and puckering your lips in a critical and rejecting expression
- Allowing your head to slump forward
- Touching your chin, cheeks, or face
- Twisting your mouth and chewing on your lips in a nervous manner
- Carrying your head forward in a chick-peck gesture
- Lifting your eyebrows in surprise or question
- Raising your forehead and creating wavelike furrows
- Frowning
- Squinting

If you find yourself frowning, avoid the people or situations that evoke that response. If you notice that you squint, check to see if the lighting is sufficient, and wear sunglasses to protect your eyes against glare. (And, do check with a doctor if you continue to squint, or develop headaches.) A positive outlook can help you overcome looking confused, unsure, rejected, angry, and fearful. Those are the responses of the helpless. You are able, fit, and secure—relaxed, happy, and even exuberant. You enjoy life, and your posture and attitude will show it.

Note: Exercising is not grimacing. You will notice that there are directions for creaming your face before almost all of the exercises. Be sure to follow that direction and apply the cream to your face. Follow this advice and avoid bad facial habits.

Now you know who your enemies are and some of the things you can do to avoid or conquer them. Be aware that you must be vigilant to stop the aging of the skin *as soon as possible*, for your skin changes as you mature. It has certain properties at one age that might disappear several years later. It renews itself, but the glands and the hormones and even the ability to renew itself change. You have to know your skin, so you can be on guard.

Your Skin Calendar—How Aging Shows on the Chin, Neck, and Shoulders

Twelve to Twenty-two

With the onset of puberty, the hormonal balance in the body changes. Many teens notice that their skin is oily, and their pores become enlarged and the blemishes may produce infections.

Some teenagers overtan their skin because tanning seems to decrease oiliness. The destructive effects won't show for a while, but excessive exposure to the sun in early youth can start some bad patterns that will produce wrinkles later on in life.

Twenty-three to Thirty-eight

Early signs of aging should not be ignored. Pores may look more refined, and usually there will be fewer blemishes (this indicates a slowdown in oil secretion). Skin should be strong, taut, and resilient.

During these years avoid sunburn and protect your skin from heat, wind, and cold. Toward the end of this period your face may seem ruddy and you might notice small lines around the eyes and a slight loosening of the skin under the chin. It is time to start a program of facial exercise and to keep your mineral spray (see p. 20) and moisturizer with you at all times.

Thirty-nine to Fifty

This is the transition period in which the effects of oversunning or rough treatment you have given your skin over the years will become evident. Your skin will need more attention now; it is rougher, thinner, and less translucent. The fat pads under the skin are thinner, and the decrease in natural skin oils means the skin has less protection. During this period your skin might become sensitive and easily irritated.

The skin on the eyelids and around the mouth, jaw, and chin might sag, and the blood vessels under the surface might be noticeable. You will now need to spend more time caring for your skin and protecting it against sun, wind, and extremes of heat and cold.

You'll need to develop an exercise program and stick to it to make this period of your life last as long as possible. You might want to reconsider some of your grooming habits and change the creams, makeup, or grooming aids you have been using.

Over Fifty

Your skin is now probably dry/dehydrated, and easily irritated. At this time, beauty habits practiced during a lifetime will reap benefits of heathful good looks. You will have to take extra care in cleaning your skin because pores become blocked very easily and your skin tends to be thin and rough.

If you have extensive wrinkling and sagging, all the natural folds and depressions of your skin will be exaggerated. Your lips might become thin, their outlines blurred. However, exercise is just as effective at this time in life as at any other. If you adhere to a facial exercise program, you can restore some of the vitality to your muscles and skin.

Learn to take special care of the skin on your neck and shoulders, and practice maintaining a posture that is both erect and graceful. You can still look beautiful at this or any age.

You are never too young to learn how to take care of your precious skin, and never too old to repair it because your skin can be improved at any age. The skin is the largest organ of your body, and it is an organ that is constantly renewing itself. Billions of cells grow, mature, and die on your skin surface. You must provide the nutrients to help them grow, the protection to keep them healthy and working, and the cleansing to rid your body of the cells when they die.

Rejuvenation Through Exercise

The skin is composed of many, many layers of cells. Among these layers are oil glands and fat cells. The fat cells form a soft cushion, and the oil glands work to clean, lubricate, and protect the skin so it will be soft, elastic, smooth, and glowing.

As we have seen, the skin is attached to the muscles by connective tissue. In youth this tissue is strong and forms a secure bond between the skin and muscles. If you drag or pull on your skin, though, you will eventually weaken the connective tissue. Harsh or forceful pressure can damage the globulelike cells and harm the texture of the chin, neck, and shoulders.

Exercising is not pulling, rubbing, or moving the skin in an undirected manner. When you exercise, you move the skin and muscles in unison so they work together as a unit. As the muscles grow strong and plump, the increased circulation that is encouraged will feed and renew the skin as well as the underlying muscles. The special exercises in this book are designed to keep the connective tissue intact.

All these exercises will firm and tone without stretching—*but you must follow the directions exactly*. If you do this, you will notice that not only your skin but also your gums, arms, neck, muscles, veins and even your eyes will seem to glow and be more alive.

Minutes to Beauty

The exercises, formulas, and the quick-working tips in this book will help you avoid all the skin agers and the enemies of a beautiful chin, neck, and shoulders. The suggestions here are designed to help you break your bad habits while replacing them with good habits. It is a natural, easy-to-master program.

Facial exercises are just as effective in tightening and strengthening the muscles of the face as body exercises are in firming the body. Elasticity, a glowing vibrancy, and the healthy color that indicates strong blood circulation are all components of a youthful appearance.

Nature will work for you, if you give her a chance. Only the very elderly and those in poor general health who are very thin cannot reverse some of the damage done by the sun, wind, tension, dehydration, poor diet, or the loss of muscle tone. In as little as three weeks your facial appearance will start to improve. Your skin will look smoother and fresher, and you will seem years younger.

To regain the look of youth and keep it forever, you must avoid the sun, fight dehydration, firm flabby muscles, and restore the undercushion to your skin by plumping up the stretched or weak muscles. Now that you know what you must do, here is how to do it.

PART II

The Program that Can Stop Time

Before You Begin

This section includes dozens of exercises developed to treat soft and sagging skin in specific areas. Read the directions carefully, perform the exercises, and soon you'll see a more youthful reflection in your mirror, a look that can remain yours forever.

The fact that muscles can develop, and skin can replenish itself, is nature's miracle. You can take advantage of this process to develop your muscles and fill out, firm up, and tighten the skin in the most telltale part of your body—your neck.

What Doctors Say

Many doctors I have worked with have asked me to provide special exercises for one or more of their patients. Doctors appreciate the rejuvenating effects of exercise, but they are often unable to spend the time teaching patients who could profit from facial exercise.

Dr. Willibald Nagler, who is chairman of rehabilitation medicine at the New York Hospital–Cornell Medical Center, recently wrote that* "Facial exercise, like all exercise, can strengthen and tone muscles—especially around your neck and mouth—and can help to prevent muscles from sagging and showing early signs of age." The only rule he insists on is that to achieve results, you *must* exercise daily.

Dr. Nagler suggests two easy and effective exercises. I've tried a version of these, and tested them with my students (they appear on pp. 36 and 45).

*This quote comes from *Vogue*, Nov. 1980.

The Muscles of the Chin, Neck, and Shoulders

In the picture you can see the muscles of that part of your face most difficult to hide, where age shows very quickly. The muscles beneath your skin support it as well as allowing movement. The bones of the face and neck and the covering of the muscles give the face its individual contours. You cannot change the shape of your bones, but you can develop your muscles to keep your chin and neck firm.

Body muscles—such as those of the arm—can be developed through exercise. The same is true of facial muscles. Every muscle is like an elastic band. Some bands are narrow and round, and some are flat and broad, almost like a stretch of elastic cloth. The *platysma* is the major muscle of the neck. It is a broad flat muscle that starts in the chin area and spreads down the throat to the shoulders. This muscle, like all muscles, is made up of round-shaped fibers grouped in bundles; each fiber activates the other fibers near it so that the muscle bundles work together. To tone and firm a muscle, you must exercise it, use it—make it work.

Examine your face, neck, and shoulders carefully. Are there any places where the muscles seem weak, flabby, or less elastic than they should be? Is the skin over the muscles dry, loose, or pouchy? Are little pouches beginning to form at either side of the mouth or near your chin? You can restore firm contours to your face in several weeks of faithful practice. With the exercises you can reverse what damage has been done, and stop or delay future damage.

Don't expect instant results, however—although many of my students have told me that they "feel" better almost immediately. It took years to develop your problems, and it will take time to correct them. But it can be done. You *will* improve the look, touch, color, texture, and vitality of your face, neck, and shoulders.

You will get another bonus from your exercises: the feeling of well-being that comes from the increased blood circulation in the exercised areas. This improved circulation will relax you, diminish the effects of tension, and even improve the texture of your hair. You'll find yourself breathing better, having more vitality and stamina, and standing so much straighter that your clothes will look much better on you.

Examine the illustration of the muscles of the neck and you'll see that muscles weave over one another and over the bones of the face

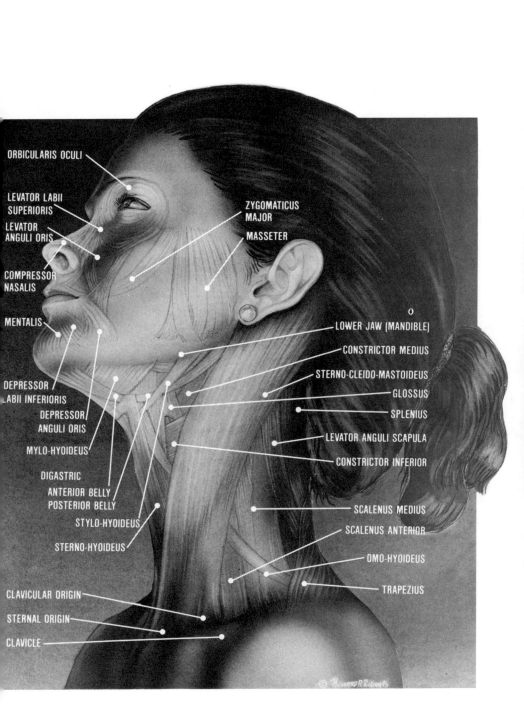

ORBICULARIS OCULI

LEVATOR LABII
SUPERIORIS

LEVATOR
ANGULI ORIS

COMPRESSOR
NASALIS

MENTALIS

DEPRESSOR
LABII INFERIORIS

DEPRESSOR
ANGULI ORIS

MYLO-HYOIDEUS

DIGASTRIC

ANTERIOR BELLY
POSTERIOR BELLY

STYLO-HYOIDEUS

STERNO-HYOIDEUS

CLAVICULAR ORIGIN

STERNAL ORIGIN

CLAVICLE

ZYGOMATICUS
MAJOR

MASSETER

LOWER JAW (MANDIBLE)

CONSTRICTOR MEDIUS

STERNO-CLEIDO-MASTOIDEUS

GLOSSUS

SPLENIUS

LEVATOR ANGULI SCAPULA

CONSTRICTOR INFERIOR

SCALENUS MEDIUS

SCALENUS ANTERIOR

OMO-HYOIDEUS

TRAPEZIUS

© Howard R Roberts

and neck to support the jaw and the movable joints. The muscles are attached by thin anchors of very tough tissue—the tendons—and seem to form a supportive net; this net allows movement, but keeps everything in place so that the effect is one of firmness, not immobility.

The exercises and massages presented here stretch and relax the arteries, veins, lymphatic system, and nerves as well as the muscles. But do not depend on the exercises alone; you must stop any degenerative habits—grimacing, dragging the skin, starving it by failing to provide proper nutrients and water, dehydrating it by allowing excessive evaporation of body fluids, and depriving yourself of the vital sleep and cleansing breaths that are needed for muscle building. Remember, everything works together.

The Best Time to Exercise

Morning, afternoon, evening—even the middle of the night—whatever time is most convenient and best for you is the best time to exercise. The only cautions are that you should not be fatigued when you exercise, and you should cream your face beforehand if creaming is specified in the exercise directions.

Many people like to exercise before retiring because they find it relaxing. Others exercise in the early evening, and follow the exercises by a short rest period or nap of about twenty minutes. They say that this refreshes them so that they really enjoy dinner or an evening show—and look better, too.

Magic Mineral Water Spray

If there is a secret beauty potion, it is water. Mineral water can help your skin look, feel, and stay youthful. I recommend spraying the face before exercising and before applying any makeup or cream. You can also give yourself a delightful pickup during the day by spraying your face and neck in the same way that you mist the leaves of a plant.

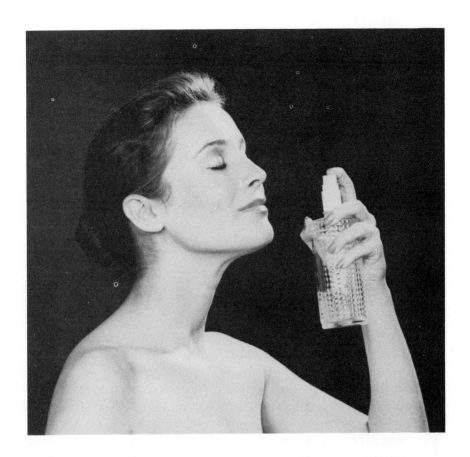

You can use a small glass bottle to store your mineral spray, you can carry it with you. You'll find that spraying your face not only freshens your skin but also makes your makeup stay on hours longer. Misting also makes breathing easier. Many dry rooms need humidifiers, and the spray will release a fine mist into the air.

Here is how to make a mineral water spray:

- Select a glass spray bottle. If it has been used as the container for any other liquid, you will have to sterilize it. This is done by boiling the bottle and any spray parts of metal in water for about 10 minutes, and then allowing them to air-dry.
- Mix mineral water (I like Mountain Valley brand) with apple cider vinegar in these proportions: 1 pint of water to 1 teaspoon of vinegar.
- Fill the spray bottle with the slightly acid mixture and seal securely.

Note: Use a glass bottle, *not* a metal or plastic container. The spray nozzle may be made of plastic.

Use your mineral water spray every time you think of it. Be sure to use the spray before applying moisturizer or protein cream for exercising. Do *not* dry your face after use.

This mineral water spray is ideal for setting makeup because it gives the skin a soft translucent glow while discouraging oily shine.

The Importance of Creaming

The directions for many of the exercises in this book tell you to cover your face and neck, and sometimes your shoulders, with cream. The cream that you use is up to you. My students usually use a "night cream" that is labeled as containing protein, collagen, or elastin. The purpose of this rich cream is to protect the upper layer of the skin (epidermis) from creasing as it is moved during the exercising. Even when you are exercising only the mouth and neck area, you should be careful to cream the upper part of the face as well. Select a cream you find pleasant to use, but remember that no product will work wonders. *You* will work the wonders through regular use and regular exercise.

How to Apply Cream

Roll the cream on the skin; do not massage it into the skin or move the skin as you apply the cream with your hands. The cream should slide onto the skin; use the pads of your fingers to glide it along. If the cream you are using feels sticky or tacky, switch to another product. Remember, you cannot use too much cream, but you can use too little—so be generous.

The covering of cream should be heavy enough to lubricate the skin thoroughly, and you should apply it smoothly and evenly. Before you begin exercising, your skin should be shiny and feel very slick to the touch.

Creaming the Face

Cream the skin under your eyes by spreading inward, from the lower edge toward the nose. When you apply cream to your cheeks, use a sliding motion up from the jaw toward the temple. Cream applied to the forehead should be spread from the middle to the temples, and upward from the nose to the brows. Be careful not to get any cream in your eyes (it is very irritating and can sting painfully).

Creaming the Chest

Guide the cream up the neck from the base of the collar bone. Then carefully cream the upper chest, above the nipples of the breasts, from midchest outward to the shoulders. Cream the armpit and the upper arm. Exercise nude from the waist up or wearing only a strapless halter or bra.

Creaming the Back

Secure your hair in a shower cap or pin it securely before you cream the back of your neck. Spread the cream over the upper shoulders, reaching down as far as you can (this reaching is a good stretching exercise).

Use Gloves If You Wish

Some people have a problem with "slippage" while doing the exercises in which you must hold one part of your face still manually while exercising another. If you have this problem, or if you are more comfortable, you can wear clean white cotton gloves on your hands during these exercises. The gloves will enable you to get a slip-free hold on the muscle and skin tissue. Slippage is to be avoided because stretching or dragging the skin away from the muscle tissue is damaging.

Taping Away Grimace Lines

Taping the face discourages grimacing and allows you to become more aware of how you habitually use your facial muscles. The tape I prefer is Micropore Surgical Tape. Clean your face and leave it uncreamed. Then:

1. Cut a strip of tape long enough to cover the wrinkle you want to erase.
2. Gently move the skin away from the wrinkle.
3. Place the gum side of the tape directly on the wrinkle.
4. Allow the tape to remain in place at least 30 minutes. (It can be worn as long as 3 hours.)
5. Place one hand on the middle of the stuck tape while carefully peeling the tape away from the edges. Avoid pulling the skin from the underlying muscles (careless pulling can stretch the skin—just what you want to avoid).

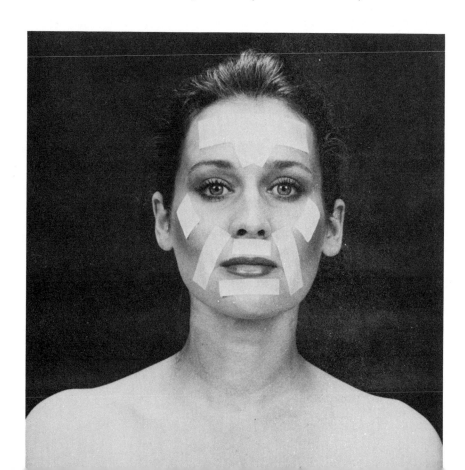

Remember to avoid eating, talking, or smoking while your skin is taped. Wear the tape as often as possible, but do not expect to see results instantly. It will take several weeks to erase the results of years of grimacing.

Note: If you experience skin irritation or find the taping uncomfortable, discontinue immediately.

General Directions for Exercising

The directions for each exercise must be followed exactly every single time you exercise, for success can only be achieved if you exercise correctly. A missed day or an occasional error will not retard or reverse the benefit of the exercise, but if you skip several days or fall into a pattern of practicing incorrectly, you will negate much of the benefit.

If you exercise twice daily for at least three months, you should see remarkable results. It will take that long for your muscles to become strong and elastic. Once your muscles are toned properly, a maintenance program of every-other-day exercise will be sufficient to keep your face, neck, and shoulders at their firmest and smoothest. If you must omit the exercises for a week or two every three or four months, no harm should be evident.

If you wish, you can divide your series of exercises into two or three five-minute sessions that can be worked into your daily routine.

As you flip through the exercise section of this book, you'll notice that one or two problems are usually treated with each exercise. After studying your face, neck, and shoulders to discover your own special problems, you may decide to concentrate on those problems that are especially bothersome to you. Happily, as you solve those problems, you will probably notice benefits in other areas.

There are two points to remember before you start your personal exercise program:

- Nature works slowly—but surely. If you are in the fourth or fifth decade of life, you may need to exercise several times a day for several weeks in order to see results. If you are quite young and beginning these exercises as a preventive measure, only occasional exercising may be necessary.

• Notice that the neck exercises also affect the cheeks, eyes, and forehead. You'll be delighted to see the many side effects of exercising, such as better color and a more graceful posture. Some people have found that these exercises even reduce the pain of headache.

For each exercise, a certain number of repetitions is specified. It is important to repeat the exercises for the specified number of times. At first, while you are mastering the exact position of each exercise, it might take you fifteen to twenty minutes or even longer to complete your exercise program. Once you become familiar with all the hand and facial positions, however, you'll be able to complete your exercise program in a much shorter period of time.

The directions for each exercise tell you how to position your fingers, mouth, or other part of your face and neck. Try to follow these directions as closely as possible. When the directions indicate *relax,* drop your hands and try to relax all your facial muscles. This relaxing is important; it prevents muscle strain.

Basic Rules for Exercising

Here is a list of basic rules for exercising:

1. *Always apply a lubricating cream* to your face and neck and shoulders when the note under the exercise title indicates that cream is needed. Do not exercise without the cream—even once.

Leave the cream on during the entire exercise period; you can even allow it to remain on your face and neck after exercising if you take a short nap. However, do not leave the cream on overnight, because if allowed to remain on your skin so long, a thick coating of cream can clog the pores. If you carefully remove the thick cream with soap and water, enough will remain to act as a lubricant and will not clog the pores. The cream will also help to carry away wastes that come from your pores, or were on your skin, or even dead skin. Your face should be cleaner and your skin in better condition after each exercise period.

2. *Breathe naturally* while you are exercising. If you have difficulty in breathing, turn to the special "cleansing breath" exercise (p.

70). These exercises will help you breathe better so that you can concentrate on the positions of your facial muscles.

3. *Always spray your face* liberally with mineral water before applying any cream or pre-exercise lubrication. Do not dry; apply the cream to your still-moist face.

4. *Exercise at least once a day* (twice a day is better) in the beginning. After each exercise is completed, relax your face until the "worked" muscles are completely at rest.

Some exercises require a resistance or counterforce. This should be a strong, firm, and slow force, as indicated in the directions.

5. *Use a mirror* while you are learning your exercises to ensure that you are following the directions as exactly as possible. After these exercises are part of your established routine, periodically check yourself in a mirror while exercising to be sure you haven't fallen into any bad exercise habits.

6. *Never exercise with a dirty face.* Don't put the lubricating cream on over your makeup or over the day's grime. Wash your face before spraying with the mineral mist and covering with the cream.

7. *Slow and steady firms the face.* During the first weeks of exercising avoid overdoing or straining your weak muscles. Consistency in exercising is better than extra effort. This is especially true during the first weeks of the program to firm your neck, jaws, and shoulders.

8. *Concentrate on each exercise* and each movement as you are doing it. Think about the placement of the hand, try to visualize the muscle working, bunching, gathering, smoothing, and growing strong. Visualize the oxygen- and nutrient-loaded blood flooding the muscle and encouraging it to become strong and round and firm.

You are about to embark on a great adventure: you are about to turn back the clock and firm and build your muscles through exercise. Used together with a program of breathing, good nutrition, and moisturizing (by misting and drinking water during the day), this exercise program can stop the ravages of time. Good luck, and have fun. Beauty is to be enjoyed, and there is no real beauty without good health and kind thoughts.

Developing a Personal Program

Wash your face carefully, do not pat dry, spray with mineral water, and apply cream lavishly. Then pin back your hair or tuck it under a shower cap. Now comes the most difficult part. Go to a well-lighted mirror and look at your face: study your chin, neck, and shoulders. Are they firm? Where are your problems? Touch the areas that seem soft and saggy.

Place your hands on the side of your jaw and urge the skin upward and outward. How do you look? Do the years seem to vanish? Place your hands on the sides of your neck and repeat the action. Now sit straight and tall; notice how much better your shoulders look when you sit up. Raise your arms so your elbows are almost at shoulder level, and then bring them back so that they almost meet in the middle of your back. Notice how the skin of your chest is stretched and how the entire shoulder area is lifted.

Get an old picture, or make a sketch of your face, neck, and shoulders, and place a mark on the areas that you want to firm. You have the power to firm and tone all the muscles in your body—including those in the neck, chin, jaw, and shoulders.

As you look through this book, you'll see many exercises for the chin, jaws, neck, and shoulders. Notice what areas and problems can be helped by each exercise. Then select the exercises and activities designed to solve your specific problems and to make you look your glowing and youthful best. Combine these exercises into your own personal mini-program.

All the muscles of the face and neck work together, as you work one set of muscles, you are probably also firming others. Any and all exercises help—but only if they are done correctly.

Creating Your Own Mini-program

What do you dream of? A firmer jaw? Smoother, fuller, more kissable lips? A neat chin? A graceful firm neck? You can realize any of these dreams by directing your exercises to that area. The following are lists of exercises that will form a mini-program for maxi-success. You can use these groups of exercises with any other exercises in the book, and you can use them in any sequence you wish. The important thing is to follow the directions on each exercise.

If your lips and chin are the areas you most want to rejuvenate, then you should combine the lip exercises (which will take five minutes), with the chin exercises (an additional five minutes) for a ten-minute personal program. Or you can spend five minutes on each of the four beauty areas for a total of twenty minutes a day, and thus create an intensive YouthLift program of your own.

Jowls
(Contouring the sides of the face, the jaws, and the area just under the jaw)

(a) Jowl-less

(b) Double-chin Disappear

(c) Great Neck

(d) Neckline

Combine for a total of 5 minutes of exercise.

Lips
(Full, round, soft, youthful, kissable lips)

(a) Kiss-ercise

(b) Happy Mouth

(c) Great Lips

(d) Upper Lip

Combine for a total of 5 minutes of exercise.

Chin
(A neat, smooth chin, delicate but firm)

(a) Chin Stretch

(b) Tongue-Chin

(c) Book-Chin

(d) Chin and Neck Areas

Combine for a total of 5 minutes of exercise.

Throat
(A smooth throat area, graceful neck, and jaw)

(a) Chin-Chin

(b) New Neck

(c) Knead Neck

(d) Hands and Neck

Combine for a total of 5 minutes of exercise.

Mixing and matching is the key to selecting the exercises that are just for you. Remember, you can do a great deal to speed up results by constantly combating your skin's enemies—weather, bad habits, dehydration, poor diet, and stress. Learn to fight these enemies at the same time that you are following your mini-program of exercise.

The All-Man Program

Actors and politicians are not the only men who are concerned about their looks today. In these high-pressure times when the competition for upper-management jobs is fierce, every man is concerned about looking as young, vital, energetic, and healthy as he can. One way of ensuring that youthful look is to maintain a firm jawline and neck. In their thirties many men notice that their necks are losing tone; the condition gets worse in their forties. Men can lift, smooth, tighten, and firm their necks—go down a collar size and recapture their youth—even more easily than women because men build muscle tissue easily when they exercise the right way.

The following exercises were designed just for a man's neck and jaw. Select any one of these, or do several in combination. Start with about four different exercises that can be completed in about ten minutes. Then experiment and master all of these easy exercises so that you can alternate them. Become jowl-less and recapture your youth.

The special Man's Program:

Round Cheeks	Neck-cersise
Jowl-less	Neck Culture
Chin Push	Bathtub Neck Straightener
Double Chin Disappear	Tummy Tightener

Follow the creaming instructions before exercising, and follow all the directions for each exercise exactly. You'll soon be on your way to a firm, square, masculine jawline.

Specific Exercises for the Face and Chin

These exercises firm the muscles and tissues of your face in the areas where the signs of aging so frequently occur.

Round Cheeks
(to smooth and firm cheeks and firm jawline)

Cream the face and neck before doing this exercise.

Note: This exercise is most effective when done slowly to the count of 10.

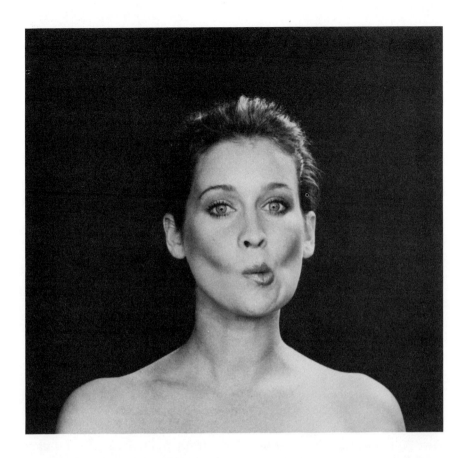

It is hard to picture this exercise exactly because individual mouths and cheeks give different effects. Both the jaw and the mouth will move when you are doing this exercise. The pull to one side of the face will cause a stretching and then a flexing of the muscles on the opposite side of the face.

1. Close and pucker or purse your lips.
2. Moving both your mouth and jaw, pull your mouth as far to the right as possible.
3. Create a suction in your mouth so that your cheek is sucked against your teeth on the left side of your mouth.
4. Using your facial muscles, pull the flesh of your cheek to the right as much as you can, keeping it against the teeth.
5. Hold for the count of 3; relax.
6. Repeat the exercise, alternating sides, until each side of the face is stretched against the molars 5 or 6 times. Do not clench your teeth.

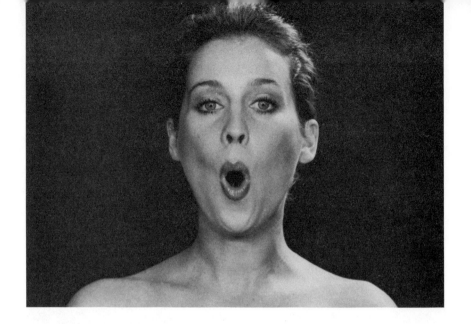

Oh! Cheeks
(to firm sagging cheeks)

Cream the face and neck before doing this exercise.

You will have to steady your face with your hands for this exercise, so you might want to wear cotton gloves. Do not allow your skin to slip. Place your hands on the sides of your face. The outer edge of your hand should be firmly held against the face from outer eye to jaw. Pull outward once your hands are firmly positioned. The muscles as well as the skin should be gently but firmly urged outward and upward to smooth out the entire face. You are now ready for the activity.

1. Holding your face firmly, push your lips forward and form them in a slight pucker.
2. Say "Oh!" and be sure the smile lines from your nose to your mouth are smooth.
3. Continue holding your face taut and say "Oh" as you move your lips first to one side of your face and then to the other. Pull your lips over as far as possible to each side—you should feel a strong pull on your cheek muscle. Alternate sides, directing your mouth first to one side, holding for a moment, and then to the other, again holding for a moment.
4. Repeat 5 times on each side of the face. Then relax, lowering your hands.
5. Repeat this exercise twice for a total of 10 mouth movements on each side.

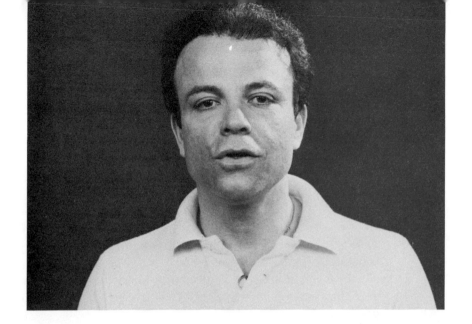

Jowl-less
(to erase pouches and sags on the sides of the face)

Cream your face and neck before doing this exercise.

This exercise will firm soft, pouchy jowls and at the same time soften or erase the smile grooves around your mouth. Since the final position must be held for an extended time, you might want to do this exercise while watching TV or listening to music.

1. Open your mouth slightly so that your lips and teeth are about a half inch apart.
2. Attempt to close your mouth, but resist by forcing one group of muscles to struggle against the closing: make hard work of the struggle.
3. As the urge to close is resisted, lift your jowls as much as possible up over your jawbone. Your jawbone should be as smooth as you can make it; try to pull your jowls up for clean jawline.
4. Say "Meow" to bring your mouth into an "O" position and stretch out the smile lines (the grooves around the mouth) as much as possible.
5. At the same time, gradually force your mouth closed.
6. Hold final position for as long as possible, up to 10 minutes.
7. End the work of closing your mouth against resistance with your mouth finally shut and your lips in a relaxed position.

Bored but Beautiful
(to tighten flabby skin and erase wrinkles
in front of the ears)

Cream the face and neck before doing this exercise.

This exercise will not make your mouth wider. The lips can be developed and filled out using the Great Lips exercise (pp. 38–39).

1. Yawn as open as possible, forming your mouth into a long vertical "O" shape. After you think your mouth is open as wide as possible—open it a bit wider.
2. As slowly as possible, close your mouth, but do not allow your teeth (molars) to meet. Close—but fight against it. Keep slowly closing and resisting.
3. After keeping up the struggle as long as possible, allow your teeth to finally meet. Hold the tension (you should feel it in your jaws and almost to your eyes) a few seconds more.
4. While holding, count to 25 slowly.
5. Gradually relax all your muscles; do this very slowly.
6. Repeat 3 times, unless the exercise leaves your jaws aching. If that happens, do it only once and try again the next day. This exercise should feel tense but not painful.

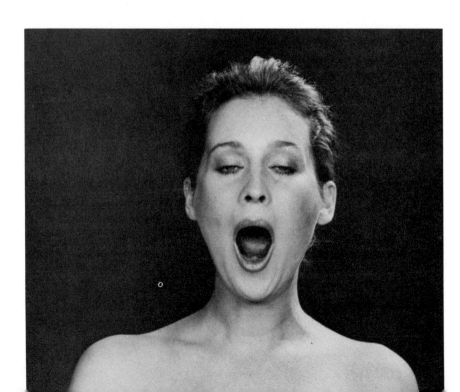

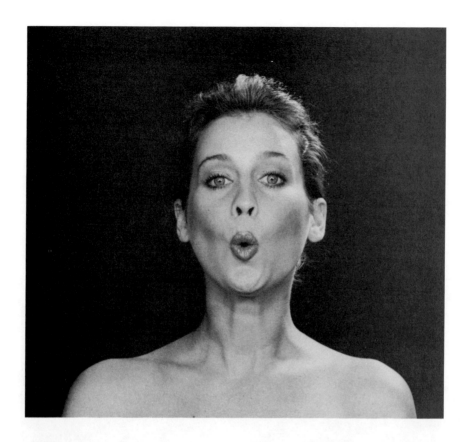

Kiss-ercise
(to firm the entire mouth area and beautify the mouth)

Cream your face and neck before doing this exercise.

Form your lips into an extreme pointed pout, pushing them out as far as possible to stretch and smooth the smiling grooves or lines that extend between your nose and corners of your mouth. At the same time, curl your upper lip upward and your lower lip downward, so that your puckered lips resemble an opening tulip. This position will stretch and erase any wrinkles around your mouth.

Don't close your lips; leave them slightly open so that your front teeth can be seen. To assume the right position, blow slightly through your lips as you whisper the word "Cheese."

1. Position your lips firmly; hold the position for a slow count of 4.
2. Relax, allowing your lips to resume their natural position.
3. Repeat 15 times.

Mouth Exercise
(to smooth smile lines and firm mouth)

Cream your face and neck before doing this exercise.

This exercise is a workout for the lips, mouth, inner cheeks, and chin.

1. Pull your lips back as far as possible. Your mouth should be somewhere between a sneer and a grimace.
2. Pull back further, baring your teeth.
3. Hold for the count of 10.
4. Relax.
5. Repeat 15 to 20 times.

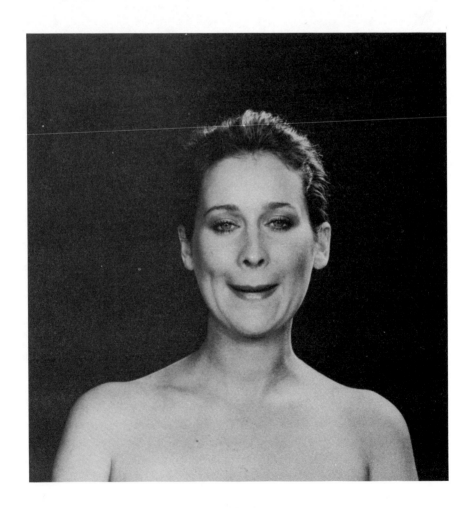

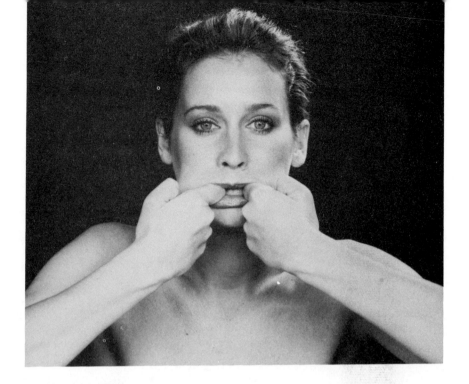

Happy Mouth
(to lift droopy mouth corners)

Cream your entire face—with special emphasis on the mouth—before doing this exercise.

This exercise will firm the outer corners of your mouth. It will strengthen your entire outer mouth area, while erasing the soft pouchy look on your lower face.

1. Insert your index fingers, up to the first joint of each hand, into your mouth, the right finger on the right side, the left on the left side.
2. Your fingers should be positioned between your lips, cheek, and gums, the nails resting against the lower teeth, the balls of the fingers turned outward against the inner mouth.
3. Keep your teeth closed and your lips relaxed and loose.
4. Using your inserted fingers, stretch your mouth out sideways as far as possible. You should feel the stretch of the fingers against the outer corners of the mouth.
5. Without moving your fingers, and while holding the corners of your mouth in the stretched position, move your upper lip inward and downward.

6. Make the movements in small steps; use the strength of the muscles to accomplish the movement.
7. Count from 1 to 10 as you move your lips, making each count a small step in forcing your lips together. You will be moving the muscles of the upper lip against the resistance provided by your fingers.
8. On the count of 10, your top and bottom lips should meet.
9. Counting backward from 10 to 1, release the muscles stretched by your fingers in small gradual steps.
10. Relax.
11. Repeat this exercise 5 times. It should be done as slowly as possible.

Great Lips
(to make lips soft, round, full, firm—kissable)

Cream your face before doing this exercise.

If your upper lip has a tendency to wrinkle, this exercise will help to prevent or erase the wrinkles.

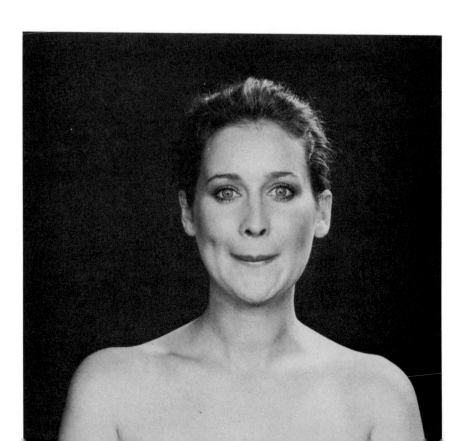

1. Pull your upper lip down over your teeth slightly. This should smooth your upper lip, which should be flat against your teeth.
2. Purse your lips—still holding your upper lip flat—slightly but firmly. A good way to do this is to say the word "Purée."
3. Lift the corners of your mouth in a tiny smile.
4. Curl the corners of your lips up as far as possible, and as you do, you will notice that the activated muscles lift your face slightly.
5. Solidify the smile by firming and tensing the lines that run between your nose and outer corners of your mouth—the smile grooves.
6. Try to make this area move upward. Control over the muscles in this area will do wonders.
7. Holding this flat-lipped, slightly smiling position, squeeze firmly, tightening and tensing the upper lip area. Hold the squeezed position for the count of 3.
8. Relax.
9. Repeat 15 times.

Grooves Away
(to plump the smile grooves)

Cream your face and neck before doing this exercise.

The smile grooves form very early if you have prominent teeth, or if there is a long distance between your nose and mouth. But don't stop smiling! Instead follow these steps:

1. Inhale through your nose in short little sniffs. Take 7 quick little sniffs and your lungs should be fairly full of air.
2. Purse your lips to whistle position.
3. Fill your cheeks and the area between your upper lip and teeth with air.
4. Exhale the 7 little sniffs through your whistle-shaped lips.
5. Relax.
6. Repeat 5 times.

Mouth Uplift
(to achieve a younger, happier expression)

Cream your face and neck before doing this exercise.

As we grow older, our muscles grow weaker—if they are not exercised. As they weaken, the mouth sags and the corners droop. When this happens, deep lines extend downward at the corners. In the following exercise you will use your hands to strengthen your mouth. This exercise will not make your mouth larger. On the contrary, it will help to contour your lips and correct your "poorly shaped" mouth.

1. Insert the little finger of each hand into the corners of your mouth. Form your fingers into little hooks.
2. Tighten the muscles of your mouth and keep those muscles firm and tight.
3. Pull outward on the corners of your mouth with your fingers, while resisting with your mouth muscles.
4. Pull with your fingers and resist with your mouth, to the count of 5.
5. Relax; remove fingers from your mouth.
6. Repeat 5 times.

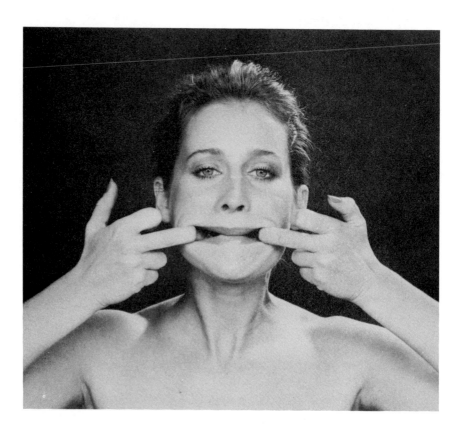

Upper Lip
(to erase tiny feather wrinkles)

Cream your face and mouth area for this exercise.

As you age, your lip area thins; this exercise will work and stretch and fill the muscle on the upper lip.

1. Place the tip of the middle finger of one hand on the tip of your nose. Hold it firmly, but do not push up. As you hold your nose, breathe naturally, through your nose.
2. Bring your closed lips down as far as possible; with the lips shut, pull down on the lips.
3. Use your other hand to help pull down on your upper lip; hold your lip under your nose. You will be able to feel the muscle stretch as your upper lip is pulled partially by your hand and partially by your own muscles over the front teeth.
4. Hold for the count of 5.
5. Relax muscles and drop hands.
6. Repeat 10 times.

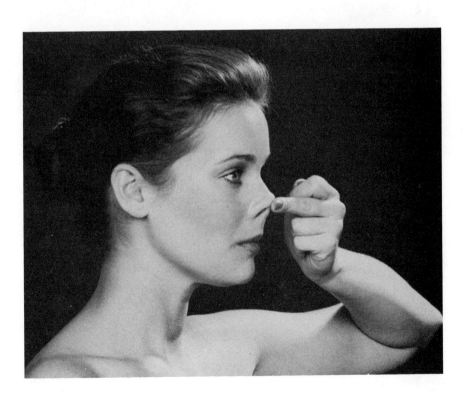

Chin Stretch
(to develop a new wrinkle that is antiwrinkle)

The cushion of muscles that covers and rounds the chin is a group of muscles that are usually involuntary. They can be moved, however, with practice and with concentration when the teeth are firmly set, though they do not respond naturally to facial gestures.

Close your mouth and place the fingers of one hand on your chin. Using your muscles only, pull your chin up as far as possible. Visualize your chin touching your upper lip. Then roll your lower lip in your mouth over your teeth as you stretch and exercise your chin. You should sense a pulling motion in your neck and actually feel your chin move up, under your fingertips.

Chin Push
(to chisel your chin—a muscle-maker exercise)

1. Form your mouth into the Great Lips position (see pp. 38–39).
2. Place the fingers of both hands—one set over the other—on your chin.

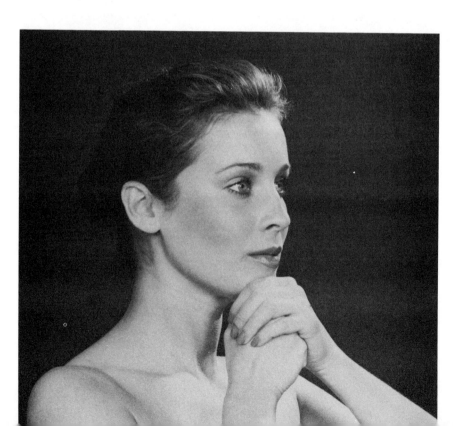

3. Press your chin back firmly with your fingers while resisting with your chin and neck muscles.
4. Continue the struggle—pressing and resisting—for the count of 3.
5. Relax.
6. Repeat 25 times.

Double-Chin Disappear
(to remove the soft underchin—fast)

Cream your face and neck for this exercise.

A long bench or a firm narrow bed is needed for this exercise. Lie flat on your back with your knees flexed and feet flat on the bench or bed. Place your shoulders even with the end of the bench so that your head hangs over the end of the bench, face up. Your shoulders and back should not move while you are doing this exercise. Your arms should be relaxed and at your sides.

1. Lie with your head hanging over the bench, your mouth in a normal, relaxed position, teeth and lips gently closed.
2. Lift your head, using your neck to raise it to normal position. Do not raise your shoulders or bring your chin down toward your chest.
3. Bring your lower jaw and teeth forward and over your upper lip and teeth. This will give you a strong "underbite" position. Keep your lips relaxed.
4. Pull your chin muscles up as high as possible by pointing and stretching your chin upward. But keep your head horizontal and up.
5. Hold for the count of 3.
6. Drop back as abruptly as possible in one fast movement, keeping your jaw forward as your head falls back. You'll feel your neck muscles working against the resistance of your jutting jaw and pointed chin.
7. Release mouth; relax.
8. Repeat 5 times. Work up to 20 times.

Note: Done twice daily (morning and night), this exercise will get speedy results.

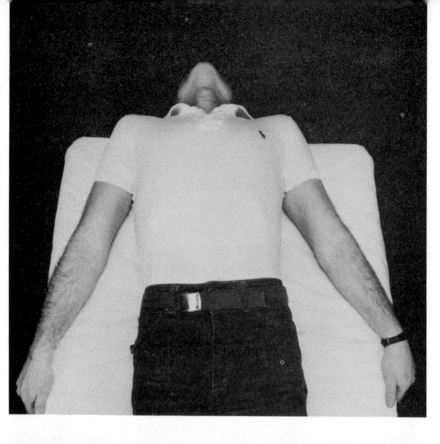

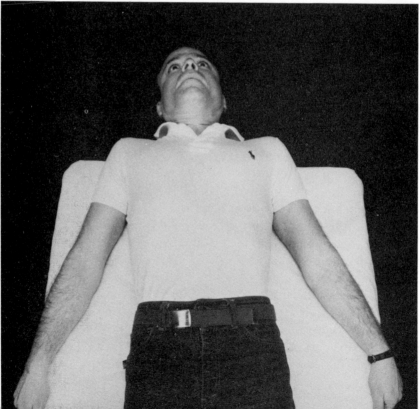

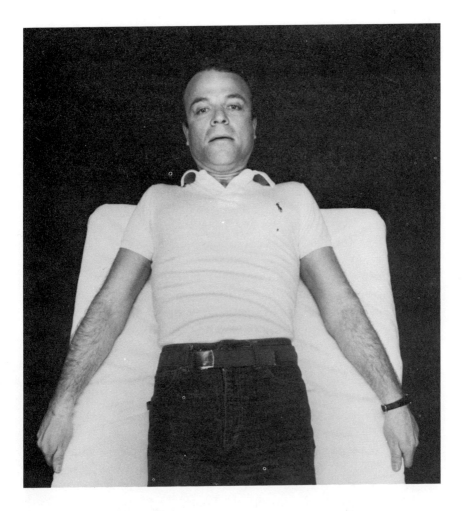

Resistance Exercise
(to fight sagging chin and slack neck muscles)

Cream your face and neck before doing this exercise.

1. Rest your elbow on a firm surface.
2. Place the heel of your palm under your chin.
3. Rest your head snugly against your hand.
4. Try to open your mouth by pushing down on your hand; use your neck and chin muscles to press against the resistance of your hand.
5. Press and struggle against the resistance.
6. Relax.
7. Repeat 15 to 20 times.

Book-Chin
(to tighten and firm chin)

Cream your face and neck before doing this exercise.

A book is ideal for providing the firm resistance used to strengthen muscles in this unique exercise. The exercise works most effectively with a hardcover book.

Note: You can rest your elbows on a table for added stability when doing this exercise.

1. Place the flat surface of a book, spine side in, firmly under your chin.
2. Push the book upward against your chin.
3. Lower your shoulders so that you do not "hunch up."
4. Place your tongue firmly on the roof of your mouth, directly behind your upper teeth.
5. Pull your lower lip over your upper lip and up toward your nose as far as possible.
6. Keep your head up and forward, as straight as possible.
7. Push upward with the book under your chin; at the same time, resist by pushing downward with your chin against the hard surface of the book.
8. Hold your bottom lip over your top lip, and with your tongue against the roof of your mouth for support, press downward with your chin. Resist this downward motion by pressing upward with the book.

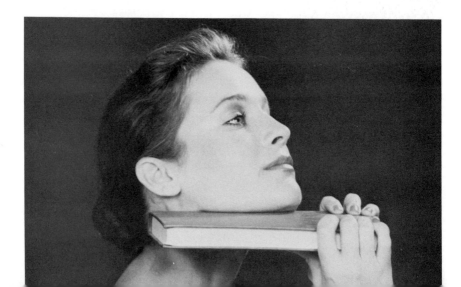

9. Hold this position for the count of 6.
10. Release pressure slowly and relax.
11. Work the book along the jawline, pressing, resisting, and counting.
12. Relax.
13. Repeat the exercise at least 3 times in each area.

Chin-Chin
(to banish turkey-neck)

The platysma is the muscle that stretches from your chin down to the base of your neck. This exercise will work that large important muscle.

1. Sit straight and keep your chin level with the floor. Your head should be poised and your teeth and lips together, but not clenched.
2. Do not move your head, but bring your lips down strongly. Draw down the corners of your mouth as much as possible (this will contract the platysma muscle from the chin to the chest).
3. Hold this position for the count of 3.
4. Relax.
5. Repeat 5 times.

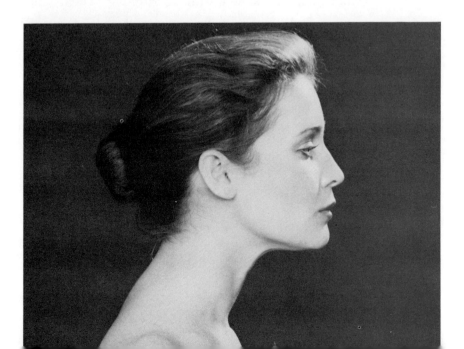

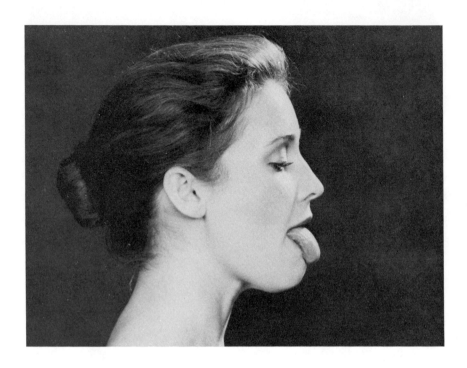

Tongue Chin
(to trim your chin, anytime, anywhere)

Cream your face and neck before doing this exercise.

This exercise can be done whenever you think of it during the day (no harm will be done if you do it without creaming). The tongue movement draws the base of the tongue forward, and contracts all the muscles that form the floor of the mouth. This is an excellent and valuable exercise because it counteracts a double chin by helping to remove excess fat under the jaw and around the neck—especially in the front of the throat. It will firm the entire neck and minimize folds of excess skin.

1. Stick your tongue out. Let it protrude downward. Try to touch the end of your chin with the tip of your tongue.
2. Point your tongue as you stretch and pull it toward your chin; then move it from side to side slightly for a moment or two. (You will become quite comfortable with this movement in just a short time.)
3. Relax.
4. Repeat 20 to 30 times, or until you feel muscle ache at the base of your tongue.

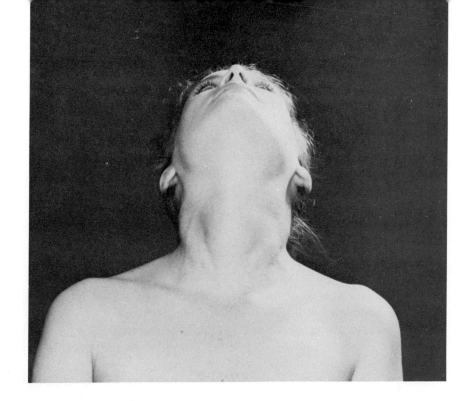

Chin and Neck Areas
(to round, tighten, and tuck the entire jaw)

Cream your face, neck, and shoulders for this exercise.

This exercise will make the muscles of the neck and jaw taut; it is very effective for tightening the area under the ears as well as in the middle of the throat.

1. Tilt your head back as far as it will go.
2. Your mouth should be slightly open and your upper lips should be brought down to cover your upper teeth. Keep covered upper teeth and lip still.
3. Stretch your lower lip down and out, exposing your lower teeth and tensing the muscles on your lower jaw.
4. Extend your jaw outward as far as you can.
5. Open and close your jaw—which should be in the position of an extreme underbite—in a chewing motion. As you move your jaw, you should be touching your lower lip to the edge of your upper teeth.
6. Chew 5 or 6 times.
7. Relax, and allow your head to move forward.
8. Repeat 5 times.

Banishing a Double Chin
(to correct posture and breathing)

Nobody wants a double chin, but before you can be successful in firming that area, you must recognize the cause of the problem. There are two causes of a double chin: collapsed muscles beneath the skin of the neck, and incorrect posture of the head and body.

To strengthen and tighten the collapsed muscles under your jaw and to erase a double chin, follow these directions:

1. Throw your head back as far as you can.
2. Try to see some point over your head, or even in back of you.
3. Place the palms of your hands over your eyebrows, interlacing your fingers in the middle of your forehead.
4. Try to raise your head from the chin-up backward position, but be careful to keep your head pressed back with pressure on the brows.
5. Slowly allow your neck muscles to win against the resistance of your palms.
6. Press forward until your chin moves forward far enough to touch your chest.
7. Repeat 5 times; relax.

Do this exercise several times a day and you will soon see a smooth, clean, firm jawline and throat instead of a double chin.

Exercises to Firm the Muscles of the Neck

If muscles are not used, they weaken and look flabby. This is true of all muscles, especially the muscles of the neck. If underexercised, your neck muscles will become flabby, even if the rest of your body is developed to the fitness and strength of a professional athlete. Remember, the face and neck often look older than the youthful body below them.

The following exercises and tips will show you how to develop the muscles that support the cheeks and round and firm the chin, jaws, and throat.

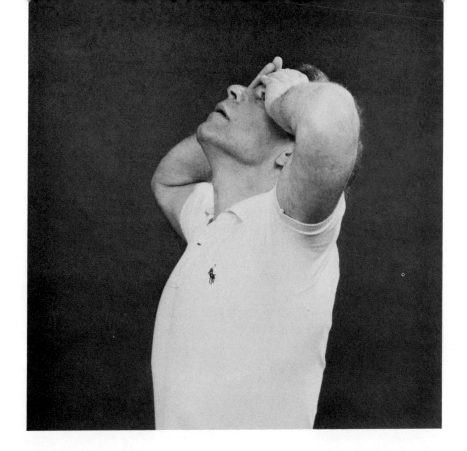

Great Neck
(to make the neck firm, rounded, graceful, and delicate)

Cream your face and neck before doing this exercise.

1. Form your mouth as you would for Great Lips (see pp. 38–39). Keep your lips pursed firmly and move the corners of your mouth upward to form a tight smile.
2. For the muscle action, press downward and outward. Cords should stand out at the front and sides of your neck.
3. Keep pressing and straining until your neck muscles are tight and the cords stand out clearly on the sides of your neck. (This exercise might not look very pretty, but remember that the *worse* you look while performing this exercise, the more effective the exercise will be and the smoother your neck will become.)
4. Hold the tensed position for the count of 3.
5. Relax.
6. Repeat 25 times.

New Neck
(to tighten and lift the entire neck for a trim look)

Cream your face and neck before doing this exercise.

Desk workers who slump or have assumed other bad posture habits will find this exercise very effective.

1. Let your head and shoulders slump forward.
2. Press your chin tightly against your chest.
3. Keep your head down, with chin tightly against your chest, while slowly straightening your backbone.
4. Straighten first your middle back, then the section between your shoulder blades, and then the section above.
5. When you can no longer keep your chin on your chest, draw back your head and neck in a strong motion.
6. Keep your chin tucked in, pressed backward into your neck.
7. As you straighten the last section of your spine, give it an added pull backward.
8. Relax.
9. Repeat 7 times, slowly.

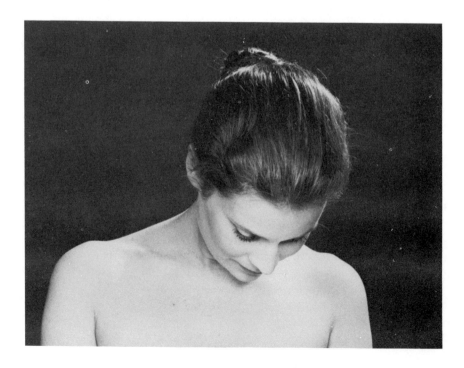

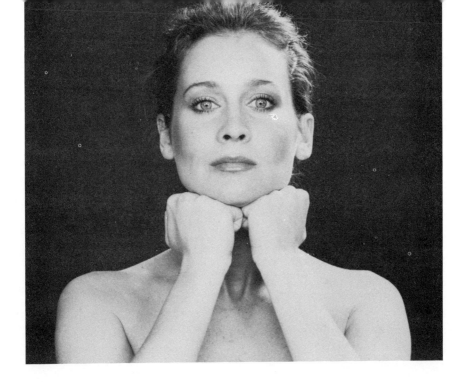

Knead Neck
(to tighten neck, using the fingers)

Cream your face and neck before doing this exercise.

While doing this exercise, think of coaxing the loose skin at the jawline toward your ears. The movement should not be too fast; little kneading steps are sufficient to press and firm. Be careful not to stretch or drag the skin in any way.

1. Form both your hands into fists.
2. Place your knuckles on your chin, right hand on the right side, left hand on the left side, with the pinkie knuckles in the center and the other knuckles extending toward each earlobe.
3. Press with a firm motion so that you can feel your jawbone beneath the skin.
4. Gradually step and move your knuckles along your jaw toward your ear; your hands will separate.
5. Knead by pressing your knuckles in firmly, then releasing and lifting slightly from the skin in almost a step motion. Press again; keep repeating the press-release motion.
6. Continue exercising as long as you can—and be as patient as you can.

Neckline
(to make the neck worthy of a diamond necklace)

Cream your face and neck before doing this exercise.

This funny-looking exercise rapidly firms the entire neck and smoothes the area where neck and shoulders join.

1. Stick your tongue out as far as possible.
2. Curl your tongue at the end so that it reaches toward your nose.
3. Hold for the count of 5.
4. Relax.
5. Repeat 15 times.

Variation: Tilt your head backward when doing this exercise. Note the additional pull.

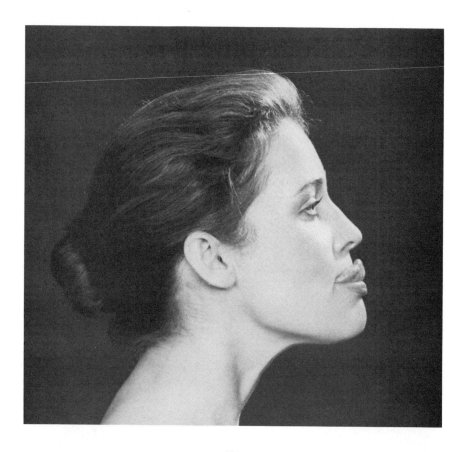

Hands and Neck
(to tighten and firm the neck muscles)

Cream your face, neck, and shoulders before doing this exercise.
Your hands will be used in this exercise, and there will be some
strong pushes. You may want to rest your elbows on a table or desk.

1. Place your left hand on the left side of your face, palm down.
   The index finger should be on the large bone just behind the
   ear, the other fingers flatly against the slight depression just
   in front of the ear.
2. Bend your head to the right, but keep your hand pressed firmly against your left cheek.
3. Firmly push your left hand upward. As you push the flesh,
   muscle and skin will move together.
4. Drop your head slowly toward your chest, still holding your
   hand securely against your cheek.
5. Raise your head to its normal position, still maintaining the
   side of the face upward.
6. Slowly drop your head backward over your right shoulder, still
   pressing the left side of your face taut and upward.
7. Drop your hand and relax.
8. Repeat steps 1–7 using your right hand to press the right side
   of your face.
9. Repeat 7 times on each side.

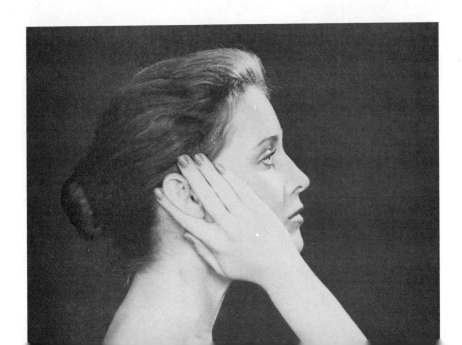

Young Neck
(after 2 weeks of this exercise, you will throw away your scarves)

It is impossible to look young if your throat is marred by loose, hanging skin. I have developed some very special exercises to firm and fill out the throat and neck muscles. For this exercise, you will need a pillow and a firm bed. Start the exercise slowly, and if you feel any dizziness, stop immediately and relax. (The dizziness results from the unusual activity and unusual position of your head.)

1. Lie on your back on a hard bed with a firm mattress. Place a firm, full pillow under your shoulders and throw your head back so that the top of your head is on the mattress.
2. Bring your head up as far as possible, and bring your chin down to your chest.
3. Once again, throw back your head as far as possible. Alternate backward and forward. Feel the great strain this exercise places on your throat muscles as well as on the muscles of the back of your neck.
4. Limit yourself to 5 movements back and forth at first. In time, you should be able to throw your head backward and bring it forward 100 times.

Shoulder Line
(to banish "dowager's hump")

This exercise will strengthen your shoulder muscles so that your posture will be alert and graceful. Do it on a very firm mattress, or use the floor, covered with a quilt or heavy blanket.

1. Lie flat on your back with your hands at your sides.
2. Keeping your arms and hands at your sides, lift your head. As you raise your head, you will feel tension in all the muscles in the back of your neck.
3. Hold your head up for the count of 3.
4. Relax.
5. Repeat 5 times.

Note: Whenever you walk with your back to the sun, the back of your neck is very vulnerable to damage from the sun's rays. (Look at the neck of a farmer, sailor, or any other outdoors worker, and you will see the kind of damage the sun can do to your neck.) To protect the back of your neck and your shoulders, apply sunscreen before going outdoors.

Neck to Floor
(to strengthen the neck
and firm and stimulate the entire torso)

You can do this exercise best on a very firm bed or on the floor (use a heavy blanket if you exercise on the floor). If you wish, you can use a small pillow.

1. Clasp your hands firmly at the back of your head.
2. Raise your head, with hands still firmly clasped, until it is about 5 inches off the bed or floor.
3. Press your head backward, simultaneously exerting pressure against your clasped hands and resisting with your hands.
4. Continue to push backward with your head as you push forward with your hands for the count of 5.
5. Relax.
6. Repeat about 5 times.

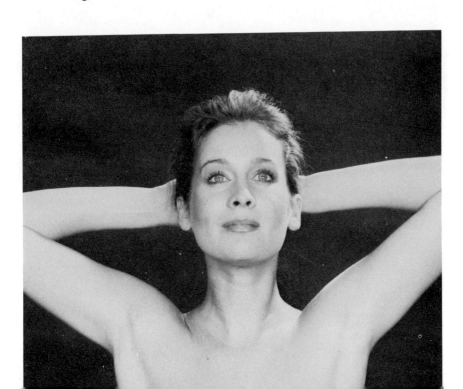

Neck-cersize
(to improve profile from jowls to shoulders)

You can do this exercise in bed if your bed is firm; if not, do it lying on any firm surface.

1. Lie on your side, resting your weight on your shoulder and hip.
2. Turn your head so that your chin is turned as far as possible toward your upper shoulder. (This movement will contract the muscles on the side of the neck.)
3. Relax and drop your head to the original position, face facing normally.
4. Turn and contract muscles, then relax; do this 5 times on each side.
5. Roll over and lie on your other side, and repeat the exercise on the alternate side of your neck.
6. You should be able to complete 10 turns and contractions immediately. Work up to about 20. (I complete up to 35 each day.)

Tongue Out
(to give the neck a good stretch)

This exercise is simple, but effective and convenient. All you have to do is stick your tongue out as far as it will go. When your tongue is fully extended, curl it up at the tip. Note how the neck lines go up and your entire throat area becomes smooth and tense.

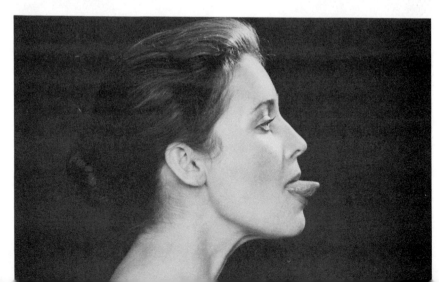

Naked Shoulders
(to stimulate the neck and shoulders—fast)

Cream your face and neck before doing this exercise.
This short, easy exercise has two parts.

I

1. Drop your head back as far as possible so that your face is parallel to the ceiling. Be sure your head is as far back as it can go.
2. Bring your bottom lip over your top lip. (You will notice a strong pull as you stretch the neck muscles.)
3. Hold for the count of 3.
4. Relax, but keep your head in the backward position.

II

5. Now stick out your tongue as far as possible.
6. Point your tongue in a downward direction as far as it will go.
7. Hold for the count of 3.
8. Relax.
9. Repeat both parts of the exercise in sequence 5 times.

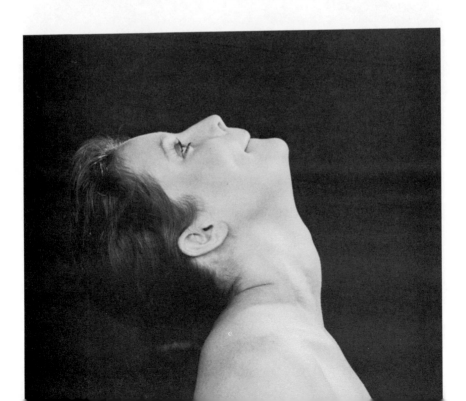

Neck Culture
(to firm the chin area and jaws)

Cream your face, neck, and shoulders before doing this exercise. Sit in front of a mirror. Your shoulders should be erect and held up and back, but in a natural position. Try to hold your shoulders and body still.

1. Drop your chin as near to your breastbone as possible.
2. Concentrate and tense the muscles of your neck, making them firm and rigid (as though you were pulling a weight), as you slowly elevate your head. Keep the muscles hard. Concentrate on making the muscles as tense as possible. Every slight movement should be an effort working against the tensed muscles.

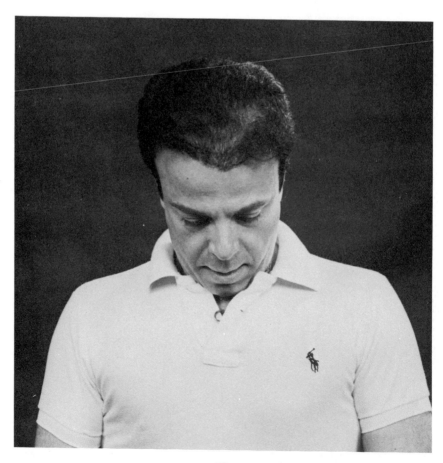

3. After you slowly raise your head, bring it backward, pointing your face to the ceiling. Keep moving backward until you can see above and in back of you—about 2 feet in back of a point over your head. Your head should be resting almost between your shoulder blades.
4. Relax, allowing your head to just lie backward, without tensing your muscles.
5. Contract all the muscles again, and move your head forward very, very slowly. Visualize lifting a weight with a forehead strap.
6. Gradually bring your head down to your chest again, keeping your muscles tense all the while.
7. Repeat this entire back-relax-forward movement 3 times. Do this exercise no more than 5 times the first week, and work up to many more times. (I have done it up to 50 times a day.)

This exercise will prevent hollows and a sticklike appearance. It will firm and fill out your neck so that it slopes gracefully to your shoulders. You'll be delighted with the results.

Tension Fighter
(to relax the entire system)

This is a neck firmer, a muscle relaxer, and for many people, a tension fighter. It can be done in an elevator, at home, at work, or even at stoplights while you are driving your car. Breathe normally when doing this exercise. Start with your head erect and facing forward.

Drop your head forward until your chin is near your chest. Then roll your head all the way around to the left, then forward, and then all the way to the right. Repeat 6 times; alternate starting left and rolling right, and starting right and rolling left.

Make believe your head is the pendulum of a grandfather clock. Drop it first over one shoulder, then over the other. First left, then up, then to the right. Repeat 6 times. Alternate, starting first over the left shoulder, then over the right shoulder.

You've been rolling left and right. Now roll back and forth. Relax your head and pull it all the way back, so you can see the ceiling directly over your head. Hold for the count of 3, then bring your head back up, and then forward and down until your chin rests on your chest.

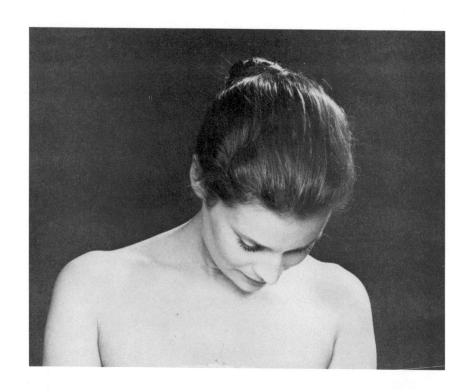

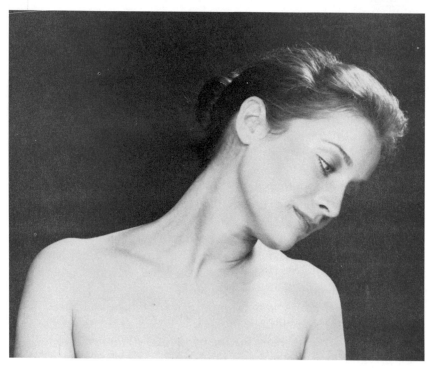

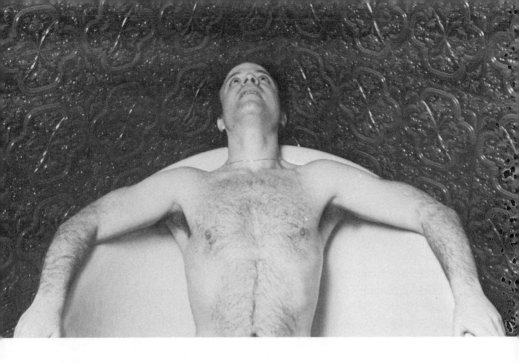

**Bathtub Neck Straightener
(to be tried only by those in perfect condition)**

Since you will be doing this exercise in the tub, creaming is not required. However, creaming your face and neck before showering or tub bathing is a good habit because the warmth and water will amplify the effect of the cream you use.

1. Relax and lie back with your head against the curving back of the tub.
2. Press your neck firmly against the tub and tense the muscles in your back, chest, and stomach.
3. Raise your upper body, resting the pressure on your neck, which is rested against the tub.
4. Your body should be balanced with the weight on your hip and the back of your head; use your arms and shoulders only for stabilization.
5. Bring your chin against your neck for additional balance.
6. Hold position for the count of 3.
7. Repeat 2, then 3 times; gradually work up to 15 times.

Note: This is a strenuous exercise. Before you begin it, be sure there is someone within calling distance. If you have any doubts or fears about your physical condition, consult your physician before you try this exercise. It is an excellent result-getter, but it is not for everyone.

"Umph"
(to tone the entire upper body)

1. Form your mouth into the Great Lips position (pp. 38–39).
2. While holding that position firmly, strain to make an "umph" sound.
3. Relax and exhale breath through your nose.
4. Breathe deeply, taking the position again; repeat several times.

While performing this exercise, you should feel the muscles in your chest, stomach, and shoulders tighten—the entire upper section of your body is being tensed and relaxed. One of my students finds this an excellent exercise for relieving tensions built up during hours of desk work.

How to Prevent Sagging Breasts

Dr. A. Christine Haycock, who is an expert on the testing of bras for use in vigorous physical exercise, believes that a more rigid bra is best during sports activities. This belief is consistent with the ideas of many French beauty experts, who insist that the breasts—especially heavy breasts—should be supported but not pulled into an unnatural position.

The directress of a large French beauty salon has the following suggestions for preserving or restoring breast beauty:

• Avoid overheating your breasts or soaking them in hot water during a bath.
• Stimulate your breasts with cold water, directed at the side of the breast with a shower head or directly from the tap.
• During your bath or shower gently stimulate the skin of your breasts with a shower mitt or friction pad.
• Apply a rich protein cream to your breasts before going to sleep every night. Using a circular motion, apply from the inside of the middle of the chest, then outward and upward to the armpit.
• Use cocoa butter (see p. 98) if stretch marks mar your breasts.

Here are some guidelines for selecting a bra:

- Try on the bra before buying it to be sure it fits well.
- Jump up and down to test if there is bouncing or discomfort.
- Be sure the bra does not limit your body motion in any position.
- Be sure the metal hooks or fasteners are covered.
- The seams should be padded or carefully finished so no rough edges can rub the delicate skin of the breasts.
- The cups should be made of cotton. Although lace looks pretty, the edges are often irritating, and nylon does not allow for enough air circulation.
- Although many women find them comfortable, some experts do not recommend underwired bras. If you like that style, be sure the wire is carefully covered and does not rub the rib cage.
- You can best tell if your bra fits perfectly after you take it off—there should be very few red marks and no deep welts on your back or sides.
- The straps should be wide and slip-proof. The weight of the breasts should not be carried by the shoulder straps—instead, the weight should be distributed over the upper body.

In-Your-Bed Exercise
(to improve breathing and complexion)

You'll need a pillow for this morning or night exercise. Place it under your shoulders and ribs so that it raises the upper part of your body enough for your head to droop backward and be lower than your chest.

1. Place the fingers of one hand lightly over your throat to feel the muscles there. As you go through this exercise, you should feel the muscles working—stretching and relaxing, growing strong, smooth, and firm.
2. Breathe in—deeply.
3. Draw your head up slowly as you count to 3 slowly.
4. Exhaling, lower your head, and relax.
5. Repeat 5 times.

Repeat this exercise as often as possible, being careful to make all the movements slow and rhythmical. This exercise is especially relaxing and pleasant when done to soft, slow music.

Tummy Tightener
(anywhere, anytime)

Stand naturally, shoulders down and relaxed, head up, but not strained. Then gradually pull in your stomach muscles. Imagine that you are trying to pull in your stomach far enough to touch your backbone. When you can pull no further, hold for a moment, and then relax. Repeat as often as possible.

This is a wonderful exercise to do while on one of those endless long lines at the bank or supermarket. Invest in your figure and posture while you wait.

Breathing and Posture Exercises

Improving Your Posture

If incorrect posture is the cause of your double chin, you will have to work at breaking some bad habits. Changing the way you hold your head, body, and arms when you sit, stand, and walk can banish your double chin. Here is a method to correct posture:

Standing: Balance your weight on the balls of your feet, hold your shoulders back and down, hold your chin forward and level with the floor. Practice this posture standing in front of a mirror. You will notice the difference immediately.

Walking: Walk naturally, with heels touching the floor slightly before the balls, but balance your weight on the outside balls of your feet. Hold your shoulders and head in the position described for standing. Your arms will move naturally as you walk—the right arm with the left foot and vice versa.

Sitting: Always sit with your buttocks all the way back in the chair and your feet and legs in a relaxed, comfortable position. Keep your back straight and sit tall with your head up. If the chair has arms, place your arms over the arms of the chair; if you are seated on a soft sofa, imagine it has arms, but rest your hands on your lap for support.

Do you read in bed? When you read, relax, or watch television, do you recline with three or four pillows propped under your head?

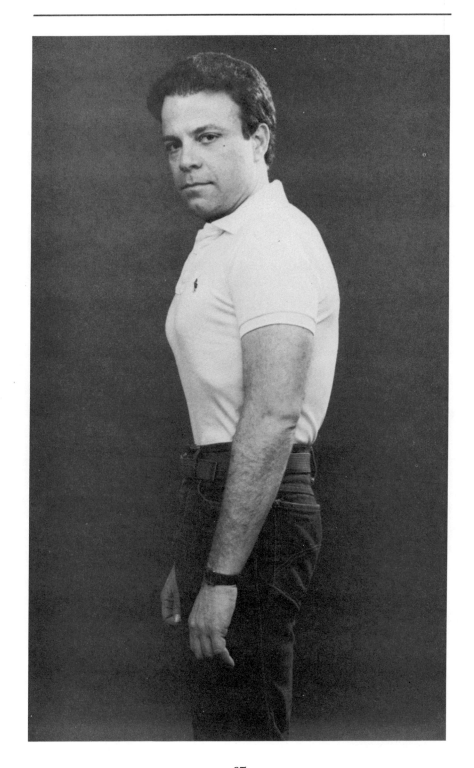

The next time you are in that position, place your hand under your chin; notice how soft the skin feels. Then sit up straight; notice how firm your skin feels now. Moral: If you must read in bed, use a slant board—a firm, hard one.

Posture is a most important factor in preventing or fighting a double chin. Exercise helps but posture is crucial.

At work, do you slouch? The worst sitting posture you can assume is to have your buttocks on the edge of the chair and your shoulders resting against the back of the chair. If you type or do other desk work, make sure your machine or whatever you are working on is placed high enough so you don't have to hunch over. When reading, don't use your thighs as a reading stand; lift the book so that you don't have to hunch over.

When you are sitting on a soft sofa or easy chair, keep your back straight and sit tall; your shoulders should be back and your chin slightly forward. When you are practicing—riding in a car or in your own home—keep your palm facing upward.

Whenever you carry heavy packages, or even a handbag, briefcase, or tote bag, carry the weight with your wrists turned so that your palm is facing forward to raise your chest. Keep your shoulders back and prevent formation of a double chin.

Getting Ready to Exercise

The best place to exercise is an open area of your home. Some people find that the living room allows them the most space; others like to exercise in the bedroom. If you live in a mild climate, you can do your breathing exercises out of doors most of the year.

When you exercise, be sure that the room or area you use is well ventilated so that fresh air can enter the room. It is important that there be enough air circulation so the air supply is constantly replenished. You may want to open your windows at both the top and bottom and to turn off any heating or air-conditioning unit in the room during the exercises. Use your judgment. The breathing exercises should not put a strain on you.

Wear loose clothing that is free of binding belts and tight elastics. A sports bra, or a well-fitted but very elastic bra with a firm cup but plenty of give in the back, might make the breathing exercises easier and more effective than tight underwear.

The next step is to expel all the air from your lungs in order to rid your body of stale air, wastes, and toxins and to make room for the new fresh air. This is an important step in the program and is a *must* before exercising and after every single exercise session.

How to Breathe Correctly

There are many exercise plans and many theories of exercise. Most of these are designed to build the muscular surface of the body. It is easier for men than for women to build the muscular system; but although women do not build large muscles, they can build agility, strength, and grace.

To firm your muscles and tighten your body, it is necessary to learn how to breathe properly. Good breathing helps you utilize nutrition and turn it into energy and encourage the growth of muscle tissue.

The system of breathing described in this book is not an unproven theory or a vague hypothesis awaiting experiment and validation. It is a complete, proven, and specific plan whose value has been measured many times. My own expanded chest measurement has increased from 37 inches before using the method to 41 inches after a year and a half of exercising. Similar results have been noted by students and others who have participated in my courses.

When you inhale, your lungs expand in size and power as the lobes fill with air. Like a balloon, your chest cavity also expands. And like a tire, the inhaled air moves, supports, and encourages all the internal organs. It also works the muscles between and around the ribs. Thus the muscles, the vascular system of veins and arteries, and the organs and glands all benefit from correct breathing.

When the lungs are used properly, they are very elastic and act in concert with the entire body to fight disease and pressures from within and without.

After you learn the basics of deep breathing, you will be able to use this breathing technique to enhance the benefits gained from the other exercises described in this book. This will include:

Breathing plus arms, hands, fingers
Breathing plus legs, ankles, feet
Breathing plus pelvis, waist, chest, back
Breathing plus shoulders, neck, jaw, head, face

At first you might find it difficult to remember how to breathe properly, but gradually your breathing pattern will change and you will find that you breathe correctly automatically. A bonus for good breathing is more energy and clearer thinking (our brains depend on oxygen, too).

How to Avoid Strain
When Doing Breathing Exercises

All the activities and exercises given in this section will help you to look better and feel more alive and energetic. But good breathing habits must be encouraged, not forced. As you perform each exercise, you shouldn't feel any strain or discomfort. About two weeks after performing this series of exercises, you should feel completely at ease with your new breathing habits and relaxed and secure as you do your exercises. Think of each exercise as an adventure in which you are discovering the strength and capacity of your lungs and body.

The exercises require concentration in the beginning. You should be aware of

- Proper breath placement
- Correct posture
- Full-lung capacity
- Exhaling and inhaling

The Cleansing Breath Exercise

Exhaling:

1. Bring your shoulders and head forward.
2. Exhale, blowing the breath out sharply between your teeth, making a hissing "sss" sound. (This action protects the throat.)
3. Expel the breath from the diaphragm upward, keeping shoulders forward and down.

This exercise is used to expel air from the lungs and to correct the habit of shallow breathing—many people never fully empty their lungs.

After exhaling and pushing out all the air you can, do the second part of this exercise—filling the lungs.

Inhaling—Inhale slowly through the nose while doing the following:

1. Stretch your arms out in front of you so they are even with your shoulders. Then raise your arms overhead and wind them first back and then forward. Your arms should be like giant windmills. Bring your head and shoulders back while filling your lungs with air. The arm and shoulder movements help to fill the lungs to their greatest capacity.
2. Breathe in through your nose. Hold maximum breath for the count of 5.
3. Relax suddenly by forcing breath out of the body. Drop hands, bend knees, open mouth and exhale to "ha" sound—force breath out quickly.
4. Repeat 3 times.
5. Relax.

Here is a summary of the entire breath-cleansing method:

Exhale stale air from lungs with quick "sss" sound from between the teeth.
Inhale deeply through nose, moving arms in a large circle and throwing head back.
Hold breath in lungs for 1 or 2 seconds.
Exhale the air sharply and suddenly from lungs through mouth with an "ah" sound. Relax, bend knees, and allow arms to fall.

As you exercise, try to visualize the old stale air leaving your body and the clean, fresh, rejuvenating new air entering your body.

If at any time you feel dizzy or light-headed, stop exercising immediately. If you smoke, this exercise might help to rid your system of tobacco toxins.

Short Controlled-Breath Exercise

This exercise should be done after the Cleansing Breath Exercise on page 70. Breathing exercises can be done any time during the day, and they are beneficial to every part of the body.

1. Place your hands lightly on your hips.
2. Inhale through your nose.
3. Hold the breath a few seconds, and open your mouth.
4. Do not allow any breath to escape from your mouth.

Note: Your mouth is held open to demonstrate that there is no contraction or stoppage at the throat. It is the diaphragm that is holding the breath within the body.

5. Holding your head and chest high, exhale, forcing some breath out between your teeth and making an "sss" sound. Keep your throat relaxed while exhaling.
6. Allow the last of the breath to escape from your body quickly, at the same time lowering your chest.
7. Repeat 5 times, taking 2 or 3 cleansing breaths between each controlled-breath exercise.

Note: During this exercise be sure that your shoulders do not rise as you inhale. Also be certain that you are really filling your lungs with air, and that it is the air that is pushing your chest cavity out and up and not just the movement of your muscles.

If you feel tension in your neck or shoulders at any time during these exercises, turn your neck from side to side several times to release the tension.

Here is a summary of the short controlled-breath exercises:

Inhale through nose while placing hands on hips.
Hold breath in lungs for several seconds; open mouth but do not allow breath to escape.
Exhale through mouth, exhaling with an "sss" sound and holding chest high while exhaling part of the air; allow chest to shrink as you rid your body of the remainder of the air.
Take 2 or 3 cleansing breaths.

Rhythmic Breathing Exercises

This is another of the rejuvenating breathing exercises. All these exercises will slowly train your lungs, ribs and muscles around the ribs and chest muscles and endow them with power—the power to control exhaling in a rhythmic manner and to pause at will.

1. Place your hands on your diaphragm.
2. Inhale through your nose—breathe in with great energy.
3. Exhale, as in the cleansing breath exercise, with an "sss" sound, allowing a portion of the breath to be released.
4. Suddenly stop exhaling and hold breath.
5. Release more of the breath through your mouth, then pause again.
6. Continue this exhale-pause pattern until all the air is expelled; drop hands to your sides.

Note: Take care that no air escapes during the pauses. Also be on guard against *inhaling* air at this time. With each pause, simply be aware of the movement and sensation of your own diaphragm. Your chest should sink a little with each short exhalation.

7. As you exhale your final bit of breath, drop your hands to your sides.
8. Take 3 cleansing breaths very quickly.
9. Relax and repeat 2 or 3 times. Since this exercise requires concentration and energy, the rest period between repetitions should be about half a minute.
10. Repeat this exercise 3 or 4 times in each exercise period over a time span of 2 weeks. Then gradually work up to 10 repetitions.

Here is a summary of the action and movements for the rhythmic breathing exercise:

Stand erect with hands lightly on diaphragm.
Exhale with an "sss" breathing from mouth to rid body of all breath.
Inhale through nose and fill lungs completely.
Exhale a portion of the breath, then stop; exhale, then stop; exhale, then stop—until all the breath is expelled.
Drop hand to sides.
Take 2 or 3 cleansing breaths, pausing slightly after each exercise.

Repeat the rhythmic breathing exercise followed by the cleansing breathing 5 or 6 times.

Tonic Breath Exercise

This exercise can be done any time of the day or night. It is both relaxing and stimulating. While doing this exercise, keep your chest as high as possible; allow it to sink only just before the last part of exhaling the breath.

1. Place your hands lightly on your hips.
2. Exhale energetically through your mouth, making an "sss" sound.
3. Inhale through your nose (moderately fast).
4. Hold your breath for the count of 3.
5. Open your mouth to establish that your neck is relaxed and there is no tension in the throat area; turn your neck to establish a relaxed feeling.
6. Exhale through your mouth very slowly.
7. Allow your chest to contract and lower slightly as the last of your breath is exhaled.
8. Allow your arms to drop.
9. Perform several cleansing breaths and repeat 5 or 6 times before relaxing; exercise twice daily.

This is a summary of the tonic breath exercise:

Place hands on hips and exhale with an "sss" sound.
Inhale rapidly through nose.
Hold chest high as you inhale; pause as you exhale.
Take several cleansing breaths.

Shoulder-Lifting Exercise

To do this exercise correctly, you must keep your body—with the exception of your shoulders—relaxed and supple. Hold your back as straight as possible.

1. Allow your hands to relax at your sides and exhale to the "sss" sound.
2. Raise your shoulders toward your ears while inhaling breath slowly into the upper lobes of your lungs. As you inhale, think about driving the air upward; you will be surprised at

the control you can exercise as you feel the air filling your upper lungs.

3. After holding the breath for a few seconds, continue to keep your shoulders high (near the ears) and exhale suddenly with a sharp "sss" sound.
4. Relax your body, bringing your shoulders and arms down to the original posture.
5. Take several cleansing breaths, relax and pause.
6. Repeat 6 times with short pauses between.

Here is a summary of the shoulder-smoothing and chest-firming exercise:

Stand erect, arms hanging at sides; exhale with an "sss" sound.
Inhale slowly, bringing shoulders up toward ears.
Hold breath 2 to 4 seconds.
Exhale with an "sss'" quickly, bringing shoulders down as air is expelled.
Take several cleansing breaths.

Some people find this exercise a great energizer!

Abdominal Pressure Exercise

This exercise firms the muscles of the diaphragm and trims the waist. It will stimulate the entire abdominal region and massage many of the vital organs and glands.

1. Standing with hands on hips, exhale to the "sss" sound.
2. Inhale through your nose with moderate speed; breathe in deeply and pressure the air to your lower lungs. Your abdomen will protrude automatically as you press the breath downward.
3. After the lower section of your lungs is filled, draw your stomach in sharply, forcing the breath up and out.
4. Take several cleansing breaths. Hold each breath for the count of 5.
5. Relax; repeat exercise several times.

Here is a summary of the steps for the abdominal pressure exercise:

Stand, hands on hips, and exhale to the "sss" sound.
Inhale quickly through nose; force air into lower lungs (abdomen will
    protrude).
Hold breath for count of 5.
Exhale suddenly and sharply through mouth to the sound "ah."
Tighten abdomen and exhale suddenly and quickly.
Perform cleansing breaths.

Posture—Rhythmic Movement

The average person does not hold her body correctly. A rhythmic walk with good posture is rare. To move gracefully and with agility, you must combine the movements of all parts of your body into an overall single motion. This walk not only looks wonderful, but is much better for your health.

You've slouched for years? It isn't too late to change. To alter your entire pattern of walking, sitting, and standing will require concentration at first, but gradually the new posture will become a habit.

To evaluate your present posture requires a hard, and sometimes unpleasant, look at yourself.

1. Pull the shades.
2. Take off all your clothes.
3. Attach a weighted string to the top of your full-length mirror. (The string will serve as a plumbline.)
4. Stand with the string passing your nose. Is one shoulder higher than the other? Does one hip protrude? Get yourself in line.
5. Turn to profile; the string should pass your ear.
6. Sit in profile. Are you really sitting straight?

Keep adjusting your posture. Practice makes grace!

Sit Up When You Sit Down
(for breathing and a dancer's graceful carriage)

It is rare to meet someone with perfect, or even good, posture. Nearly everyone slumps, and most people have acquired very bad habits of posture. Yet we all admire good posture when we see it.

Becoming aware of your posture is the first step in improving it. When you stand, sit, or walk, lead with your chest. Think: Up, firm, forward. With shoulders down, back, and relaxed.

Good posture is essential for good looks. It also helps you to look younger because it keeps your back erect. It is depressing to see how many people have bad posture. Every time I see someone who has an unmistakable double chin even though she is not obese, I know that bad posture is to blame.

PART III
Skin-Care Recipes and Techniques

Kitchen Cosmetics

This section includes more than a dozen very simple recipes for homemade cosmetics. The advantages of these recipes are that the ingredients are easy to find, very few ingredients are used in any single recipe, the preparation is simple, and—probably most important—these recipes work.

Vegetables—especially those in the cucumber family—seem to refine pores and soothe skin. Oils and oily vegetables and fruits, such as the avocado, moisturize skin and clean as well as protect it. Acid liquids and citrus fruits clean as well as stimulate the skin. Lemon, one of the great beauty fruits, has a slight bleaching effect on skin and hair. It also prevents some bacteria from finding a home on your skin surface.

Before using any of these recipes on your face or body, *test* them for allergic reaction. You can do this by applying a small amount—just a dab—on the inside of your arm or on the side of your neck. Wait at least 24 hours to see how your skin reacts before you apply the rest of the recipe. If you have any adverse reaction, don't use the preparation.

Store all leftover food-cosmetics in sealed containers in your refrigerator.

Tip: In selecting a bowl or jar in which to mix and store your homemade cosmetics, choose only glass or ceramic jars or bowls for mixing or storage. Use only stainless steel or wood as a mixing utensil. One of my students keeps a small stainless steel butter knife, a demitasse spoon, and some glass jars that have been sterilized by boiling for her cosmetics. She says that having those utensils on hand makes cosmetic-making easy and efficient.

Oatmeal Masque

This masque will leave your skin bright and fresh.

A handful (about 1/2 cup) of raw oatmeal.
Enough warm mineral water to form a paste with the oatmeal
Spread the warm paste of oatmeal and mineral water on your face and neck and allow it to dry. The paste will remain warm for a long time because oatmeal retains heat. As the masque dries and cools, it will absorb oil, grime, and wastes from your skin. When the masque is dry—in about 30 minutes—rinse it off with cool water.

This masque is clarifying but gentle enough for most sensitive skins.

Apple Cider Astringent

Keeping your skin slightly acid helps to fight infections and small blemishes.

1 part white apple cider vinegar
1 part Mountain Valley water

You can mix this astringent in a clear sterile glass jar and keep it in the refrigerator. Apply by patting on skin after cleansing; allow to dry on skin surface. Avoid splashing in your eyes.

Carrot Tonic

The carrot has many nutrients (as do most root vegetables), which makes it an excellent skin tonic. The coloring in carrots (carotene) helps your skin to withstand the sun's aging rays.

1. Purée 3 large carrots in a blender, adding as little water as possible.
2. Pat the fresh carrot juice on your skin with a cotton ball or a soft natural sponge.
3. Allow the juice to dry on your skin, and to remain there for about 30 minutes.
4. Remove with a warm-water rinse.

Cucumber Tonic

The juice of the cucumber is a wonderful stimulant for tired skin and an excellent tonic for oily skin.

1. Peel and seed 2 medium-sized cucumbers.
2. Mash or purée the pulp in a blender.
3. Pat on with a cotton ball.
4. Rinse with cool water to remove.

This pickup for tired skin is especially refreshing in the summer heat; it is also excellent for reducing enlarged pores.

Wine Tonic

Wine, like some other acid beverages, makes an excellent skin tonic and freshener. Apply it as you would any astringent or toner. White wine is best for dry skin, red wine for oily skins. Rinse with cool water to remove.

Brewer's Yeast Masque

This masque is perfect for dry, nutrient-starved skins. It softens, cleans, and closes enlarged pores.

1 tablespoon of brewer's yeast
½ tablespoon of olive oil
1 egg yolk

Mix together, blending well, and apply with a cotton ball. Allow the masque to harden for about 30 minutes. Remove with a warm wet washcloth, followed by a rinse with cool water.

Honey Face Masque

This masque brightens sallow skins. Effective on dry, oily, or combination skins, it is the perfect pickup after a busy day.

2 egg whites (reserve the yolk for the Brewer's Yeast Masque
2 tablespoons of pure honey

Blend together well. The mixture will be slightly tacky. Using your fingertips, in an upward-outward motion gently massage the masque into your skin. For best results, lie down and relax while allowing the masque to dry on your skin (about 30 to 45 minutes). When the masque is dry and no longer sticky to the touch, rinse it off with warm water.

Bleaching pack (A)

This pack can be used on the face, neck, shoulders, or breasts. Before using, be sure to test for sensitivity to lemon juice; if your skin is extremely sensitive, dilute the lemon juice with a teaspoon of water.

Juice of 1 medium-size lemon
2 tablespoons of wheat flour

Mix lemon juice with wheat flour in a glass or ceramic bowl with a wooden mixer. Apply the pack with your fingertips (the lemon juice will bleach any stains on your fingers). Allow the pack to dry, then wash off with warm water.

Bleaching Pack (B)

This pack is strong and will make freckles or dark spots vanish in a short time.

1 ounce of hydrogen peroxide
¼ ounce of wheat flour

Mix together in a glass or ceramic bowl with a wooden mixer. Apply the pack to your skin with your fingers, smoothing it gently; do *not* rub it into your skin. Allow to dry, then wash off with cool clear water. Be sure to rinse well.

Yogurt on the Neck

Plain yogurt is wonderful for the skin. It alleviates small crepe lines and evens out the pigmentation.

1. Apply yogurt to freshly cleansed neck and throat.
2. Allow application to remain on overnight.
3. Wash clean with tepid water in the morning.
4. Repeat as often as possible.

Oatmeal Bath

Here is a relaxing beauty bath that will leave the skin all over your body soft and clean. It has none of the disadvantages of a commercial bubble bath, and possesses many of the benefits of a health-spa treatment.

You will feel revitalized.

1. Place a handful (about ¼ of a cup) of raw oatmeal in the middle of a handkerchief.
2. Tie the ends securely so that the oatmeal cannot escape.
3. Steep the oatmeal package in a bowl of very hot water for about 10 minutes.
4. Fill the tub with water for your bath.
5. Add the oatmeal package and the oatmeal water it has been in.
6. Relax in the tub for about 10 minutes.

Sand Bath

If you live near a sand beach, or vacation at the beach, you can enjoy a real beauty bath. Bury your entire body—except your face, shoulders, and hair, of course—under a light covering of sand. This sand blanket is similar to the famed "Turkish bath" without the fuss or discomfort. The moist sand is refreshing and the slightly abrasive action of each particle of sand will leave your skin glowing and polished.

While your body and limbs are buried, protect your face, shoulders, and hair with a hat and a sunscreen.

Puffy Eye Compress

Red, swollen eyelids and puffy lids respond almost immediately to a compress of raw potato.

1 small raw potato, peeled
3 to 5 inches of loosely woven 2-inch gauze

Grate the raw potato with a kitchen grater. Place about a tablespoon of grated potato between two pieces of gauze. Make two gauze and potato "sandwiches" and place them on your closed eyelids for 30 minutes. Rinse off residue with cool water.

Repeat this treatment every day for several weeks for chronic puffiness; if puffiness doesn't disappear completely it will certainly diminish.

Chin-Chin Strap
(a secret weapon in the war against sags)

This device can help enormously when it is supplemented by exercise. It will whittle away soft underchin fat deposits and bring out your youthful, firm chin line. It is especially helpful for loose skin and hanging jowls.

Here is how to make a chin strap:

1. Fold a soft cotton cloth or large handkerchief in half so a triangle is formed.
2. Spray face, neck, and underchin with mineral-water spray.
3. Attach a strong rubber band to the two ends at the base of the triangle and adjust the device so that the cloth handkerchief is under your chin and is held taut by the rubber band circling to the top of your head.
4. Adjust for a comfortable but tight pulling motion.
5. Pull the handkerchief down slightly and place a small piece of plastic wrap between the handkerchief and your skin. (The kind of plastic used in bags is fine.)
6. Replace the handkerchief against your underchin.
7. Wear the device as often as possible. You can even sleep in it if you find it comfortable enough.

Note: I like chin straps made of gum rubber; however, you can fashion any number of workable devices from elastic, rubber, plastic, or stretch fabric. The important thing is that the device support your underchin with slight pressure in order to discourage fat deposits.

After-Bath Rich Moisturizer/Exfoliant

1 pint of avocado oil
1 tablespoon of sea salt

Mix the sea salt into the oil. Shake well. Spray the body or area to be moisturized with mineral-water mist. Put the moisturizer–oil/salt on a face cloth and rub it over your body. Rinse with tepid water. Your skin will feel velvety soft and smooth.

Moisturizers

Beautiful skin is soft, even-colored, glowing, slightly moist, and velvety rather than oily or dry in texture. Try this experiment to see the benefits of moisturizing (you can do it in your own kitchen). Partially fill a small plastic bag with water. Fold it, scrunch it, press it with your finger. Notice how the water forces the plastic back again—the bag becomes smooth, clear, and plump looking. This is how moisture helps to keep your skin young looking.

When the skin dries, as it does with age, the cells become less efficient at holding moisture. As a result, the skin loses some of its bounce and the outer layers appear dry. The skin also loses its translucent, light-reflecting beauty. The drier the skin, the deeper the lines that will form on it. Severe dryness may be so destructive to the skin that cracks, breaks in the tissue, and patchy flakes of dead skin appear on the surface. The skin then looks old, rough, grayish, or florid; it is no longer even colored and softly glowing.

The drying of skin starts long before its effects become visible. The drying of the skin on the face usually begins at the outer edges of the eyes and on the sides of the face. These first lines (crow's-feet) appear because the skin in this area is thin and contains few oil glands. Oil glands work to clean the pores, but also act as a natural barrier, guarding against the evaporation of precious *water moisture* from the skin's surface.

A moisturizer is a light emulsion of water and oils that protects your skin cells. Use a moisturizer under your makeup or alone; apply it at least twice a day. Never apply a moisturizer to dry skin; always mist your skin before applying a moisturizer. Get into the habit of applying moisturizer to your still-moist freshly washed face. A bonus for using moisturizer is that your makeup will go on more smoothly and will last longer with less tendency to change color.

Creams and Other Skin-Care Products

Carefully read the labels on every product before you buy or use it. Cosmetics are most frequently a combination of water, oil, and colorants with stabilizing ingredients.

Night creams are usually very rich in oils and contain less water than moisturizers. Some of the newer creams include protein substances such as collagen and elastin. These substances, produced in the bodies of living creatures, encourage the elasticity and vibrancy of healthy young skin.

Exfoliation

Exfoliation is the process of shedding the old, dead or dried skin cells from the surface of your face and neck. Have you ever looked at yourself and decided that you are wearing yesterday's face? You might well be! Skin cells die and shed easily when we are young. This process slows down as we age. These dead dry cells could be the reason your skin appears lifeless and gray.

Exfoliation can be speeded by slowly brushing the dead skin away with a complexion brush (natural bristles *only*) or by applying exfoliating rubs and peels. These rubs and peels are usually a combination of some abrasive material and a cream. The abrasive action loosens the cells and the soap or cream carries them away from the face. A more dramatic exfoliation, which will reveal fresh new skin, can be obtained under the supervision of a practiced cosmetician who uses special masques or a combination of masques and chemicals.

Since your skin is always renewing itself and the shedding of skin is continual, you can keep your skin looking fresh and translucent with new moisture-filled cells with an at-home program of brushing and masques. The exfoliation should be done at least once a week—more often for oily skin because the dead cells have a tendency to lump together and clog pores. But even dry skin needs exfoliation.

If you begin a program of exfoliating now, you will see results very soon, and you'll be delighted with the compliments you receive in about four weeks. Your skin will be free of the residue of dry dead flakes, and will have a fresh youthful glow. Make exfoliating part of your weekly beauty program.

Dry-Brush Massage
(a wonderful health and beauty secret)

Note: For this special beauty treatment, you'll need a brush of goat hair or one of boar bristles; if you prefer, you can substitute a loofa or a glove of twisted hog's hair. Do *not* use a nylon or synthetic-fiber brush or buff pad because nylon fibers can actually damage the skin. Natural fibers are smooth and rounded when viewed under a magnifying glass; the man-made materials have sharp edges.

Start the massage at your feet. Brush vigorously in a circular motion. Then gradually move up your body; do not forget the insides and the backs of your legs and arms. Don't hesitate to brush your breasts lightly, and be sure to reach the middle and small of your back. Your first efforts might be difficult, but the brushing is very stimulating. Continue brushing for between five and ten minutes.

The best time for this total-body experience is when you get up in the morning and/or before you go to bed at night. The sensation of a brush massage is both invigorating and relaxing. If possible, brush just before you bathe or shower (a shower or bath is a great follow-up because it rids the skin of loosened dead skin cells). If you cannot shower, sponge your entire body with a wet sponge or cloth.

This brush massage is a version of the "Russian bath." If you live near a spa or salon that provides a real Russian bath, treat yourself to this beauty-health experience, for it is incomparable. In a traditional "Russian bath" your entire body is rubbed and stimulated with oak leaves. The acid quality of the leaves is fabulous for the skin. And the brush massage has many of the same advantages.

- It removes the dead skin layers or flakes of dry skin.
- It cleanses the pores and encourages the body to rid itself of toxins and impurities.
- The brushing results in younger-looking and younger-feeling skin.

- The nervous system is stimulated by the skin's reaction to the brushing.
- Heightened blood circulation results from the brushing.

Caution: Avoid brushing the genitals or parts of the body that can become irritated by the friction. Do not brush so vigorously that your skin becomes red or tender; brush only as long as the sensation is pleasurable.

Your brush or loofa will collect bits of dead or dry skin with each brushing. This waste material is an ideal home for bacteria, so wash the brush with *very* hot water after each use. Cleaning your brush regularly and allowing it to dry in strong sunlight will keep it fresh and immaculate for future use.

After the follow-up shower or sponge, pat your body dry. Then spray the new fresh skin of your body with Magic Mineral Water Spray (see pp. 20–21) and rub in a small amount of sesame or avocado oil. You will be amazed at how soft and fresh your body feels—and it will stay that way with regular treatments. The Magic Mineral Water Spray and oil coating are especially important if you live in a cold or dry climate, or if you suffer from dry skin.

PART IV

About Your Body and Health

Mae West's Star Secret

We'll all miss Mae West; she was a wonderful comedienne, and she certainly livened up our language. Mae West retained her youthful, pink-white delicate complexion through her entire life. Because her skin was taut and firm, she never seemed to age. She adhered to a strict regimen all her life; she was as careful of what she did to her body and skin as she was of the exquisite clothing she wore.

Mae West's health regimen depended on cleanliness and water. Her motto—one that every woman should hang on her mirror—was: *You're never too old to become younger.*

Believing that you must be clean inside as well as outside, Mae took an enema once a week. Understanding the importance of water in staying youthful, she drank only mineral water—never water from the faucet. She was so careful that she even used bottled mineral water to wash her face.

Mae perfected a special face-washing technique that she believed kept her skin clean, protected, moisturized, and youthful. Here it is:

Wash your face with mineral water, carefully splashing away all soap or cream residue.
Combine rosewater in equal parts with mineral water and mist your face with the mixture.
Moisturize your skin carefully with a good moisturizer.
Apply makeup.

Mae West was also very careful about her diet. She ate only the freshest, most natural of foods. No additives or preservatives for her—she consumed only "health foods." Part of her health-and-beauty program involved *not eating:* Mae West fasted one day a week every single week.

We'll miss Mae, but we can profit from her beauty wisdom. Perhaps it will keep many others looking radiant into their eighties.

Circadian Rhythm

If you often travel by plane, going long distances in a short period of time, you've probably suffered from "jet lag." If you've worked at night or at an unusual time, you may have felt out of phase. Everyone has an individual body cycle. This is the complex cycle that your own system demands. Your sleep pattern, heart rate, blood pressure, food digestion and use (metabolism), the growth of your cells, your blood-cell count, kidney function, and even your rate of breathing follow a pattern. It is usually of about twenty-four hours' duration.

The pattern generally shows peaks and valleys of body functions. Some people are aware of their pattern. For instance, you might call yourself a "morning person," meaning you tend to rise early and are full of energy in the early morning. Or you might describe yourself as a "night person" who can stay up well past midnight, though you never feel wide awake until afternoon. Most people fall somewhere between these two extremes.

Your biological body clock, just like the sleep-awake pattern of all animals, makes survival possible. Even the simplest of all creatures responds to light and dark, cool and warm, by a shift in body function. Scientists believe that our body clocks are somehow linked to the process of aging. This process includes changes in hair, skin growth, and even how we use the food we eat.

Become aware of your own pattern and try to work and live within it. When do you feel hungry? Tired? When are you most alert? Plan your exercise program around the time that feels most natural, because that is when it will be most effective. You can easily determine this by exercising at different times and seeing which time of day—or night—seems most natural to you.

Sex

Yes, sex is good for you! During sexual activity increased amounts of sex hormones are secreted by the glands. These hormones enter the bloodstream and circulate to every part of the body. You've probably read or heard about rejuvenation techniques involving the injection of sex hormones—such as estrogens (female) or testosterone (male)—into the blood. Sexual excitement and arousal are the best way to get additional sex hormones.

An active and exciting sex life is one of the best prescriptions for preserving a youthful face and body. The activity, just like any physical activity, might tire you, but it also invigorates you. The glands perform better the greater the demand made on them. So sex is actually a healthy, natural way to look and be young.

New Vitamin Knowledge

Vitamin E is thought to be the leading preventive of some aging agents that attack the skin cells. Vitamin E is an antitoxin—a substance that helps your body fight negative forces that lead to degenerative diseases and aging.

Vitamins and minerals are still mysterious in their use and effect on our bodies. Many people believe that vitamins act like drugs. Linus Pauling and many other noted scientists have studied the effects of vitamins on our bodies. New information about vitamins is often in the news. You should take note of the information, but also notice how often these "wonder cures" prove to be exaggerated or to have serious side effects.

As we age, our bodies lose their ability to use certain vitamins. After a certain age—it varies with general health and inherited characteristics—our ability to reproduce healthy cells is diminished.

What does all this mean? It means that you must be vigilant about your own physical needs so you can use what has proved effective for you.

Pantothenic Acid

You've probably seen reports or advertisements that praise the properties of royal bee jelly because of its extraordinary effect on longevity. If the larva of a female bee is fed the usual amount of jelly, the result is a drone bee—whose life span is usually a few short weeks. However, if the female larva is fed extra royal jelly, the result is a queen bee—strong, fertile, and with an expected life of six to eight years. Roger Williams, of the University of Texas, has been carrying out experiments with the royal bee jelly. The jelly is very high in panthothenic acid. This has been found to have great value.

How Old Is Old—Increasing Life Span

Dr. Alexander Comfort, a leading gerontologist at the University of London and noted writer, says, "If we kept throughout life the same resistance to stress, injury, and disease that we had at the age of ten, about half of us here today might expect to survive in 700 years' time. There is no evidence that anyone has lived 700 years, so man's maximum life-span to date is far short of this intriguing potential."*

In 1927 Dr. Clive M. McCay launched a now-famous study of the effects of diet on life span. The results of the experiments were published in 1932, and were of great interest to the entire scientific community. McCay's experiments were conducted on laboratory rats. He was able to lengthen their life span by controlling their diet and intake of food. Both the growth rate and weight of the underfed rats were retarded.

Dr. McCay used deliberate underfeeding to produce a long delay in growth rate and development of the rats (which are mammals, like us), but perhaps of greater significance, his research indicated that the life span of these mammals could be doubled. Further, the periods of youth and young adulthood as a percentage of the total life span could be increased. In human terms, youth—from the ages of one to twenty—might be considered as one-fourth of a life span of eighty years; young adulthood—from twenty to forty—might be considered another fourth. McCay's research showed that these periods of vitality and vigor could be prolonged in rats—under special conditions, underfeeding prolonged their life span, and conversely, overfeeding decreased their life span.

Whether these findings apply to human beings cannot be said with certainty.

Antiaging Foods—A Way of Life

A carefully controlled diet of specified nutritional proportions is probably an important part of an effective antiaging program.

Aging—The Biology of Senescence (London: Routledge & Kegan Paul, Ltd., 1964).

Infections and bacterial diseases have been controlled through drugs. The degenerative conditions that often accompany the aging process can be partly controlled, though not completely eliminated, by improving nutrition, with the help of vitamins E and C and the minerals zinc and pantothenic acid. All evidence indicates that these are effective antitoxicants, and that they reduce oxygen requirements for healthy tissues by regulating the amount of oxygen needed to burn fats. They also help the body to use carbohydrates and proteins more efficiently.

Stretch Marks

There is, unfortunately, no way to completely rid yourself of stretch marks once you have them. The trick is to avoid getting them. Whenever you gain or lose weight rapidly, you are prone to getting these light-colored rivers. They usually appear on the sides of the stomach, the lower back, and the outer thighs. The sides of the breasts are also vulnerable.

Stretch marks can be a real problem for both men and women—they are certainly a source of embarrassment and insecurity. The following formula works to prevent and help diminish marks.

Cocoa Butter Cream
(enough for several applications;
keep in a cool dry place, sealed)

2 tablespoons of cocoa butter
1 tablespoon of avocado oil
1 tablespoon of wheat germ oil

Melt the three oils in the top of a double boiler; when melted, mix until blended. Apply to the stretch marks, rubbing across the lines.

Did You Know?

- In one square inch of skin there are over fifteen million cells, and almost twenty feet of blood vessels. There are also dozens of hair follicles and tiny oil glands and thousands of sensory cells that react to the slightest touch or change in temperature.

- Laughing increases your blood circulation, so enjoying yourself is good for your skin. When you smile, you stretch and firm about fifteen muscles in your face. In contrast, when you frown, you contract and suppress about sixty muscles. Frowning also prevents the even flow of blood to the muscles.
- "Adolescent" skin problems do not always disappear after the teens; many women in their thirties suffer from acne brought on by stress. Acne is most prevalent on the forehead, around the mouth, and on the chin—and also on the shoulders (there are more oil glands on the back of the neck and the shoulders than on the throat area). If you have a tendency to get acne on your shoulders, use an exfoliant and an astringent in that area.

A Woman's Facial Hair

We all have hair follicles all over our body. Everyone has some facial hair—and hair present in normal amounts should not be removed. However, if you have more than the normal "peach-fuzz" on your upper lip, chin, or lower cheek, it can be embarrassing. This facial hair is the result of your body chemistry. Since it might be a symptom of hormonal imbalance, before you consider any method of hair removal from your delicate feminine face, consult your doctor.

Women who have dark hair are usually more aware of their facial hair than blondes. Dark or coarse facial hair can be bleached. Waxing is a method of removal, and for most people, this method is effective for from three to five weeks.

Depilatory creams, which usually contain alkaline agents that destroy the structure of the hair, causing it to break away from the surface, can also be used. However, these chemical creams should never be applied to sensitive skin or problem skin. Chemical depilatories always carry the risk of irritation, so it is very important to test your skin's reaction to these chemicals before you apply the cream to your face. Always read the directions on any label very carefully.

Plucking or tweezing is the most common procedure for removing scattered hair on the face. Unfortunately, the new growth can be darker and curlier or more wiry hair (almost as if nature were fighting back).

Small hairs near the surface of the nostrils, or on a mole, should be clipped with small scissors. If such hairs really distress you, see a licensed expert in electrolysis. Electrolysis has been around for a long time; it is painless if done correctly, and it is very effective.

The Skin Remembers

I'm often asked about the dark frecklelike spots that frequently start to appear on the skin in the late thirties and continue to appear as the skin ages. These spots are most annoying when they are on the shoulders, chest, or backs of the hands. They appear because earlier in life—perhaps ten to twenty years earlier—you overtanned or burned your skin. These spots are sometimes called "liver spots," although they have nothing to do with the liver; they are areas of hyperpigmentation caused by hormonal changes in combination with a weakening of the skin's elastic and fat pad. The best way to avoid these spots is to avoid the sun. If you use bleach cream to fade the spots, avoid the sun because the sun will make the spots reappear—the skin does remember.

The pinpoint-sized dots of red that sometimes appear on the body are broken capillaries. They also indicate a thinning of the understructure of the skin. To prevent these red dots, avoid very hot or very cold water in your bath, and dress carefully in cold or hot weather.

Deodorant soaps, perfume, and lime (among other cosmetic preparations) can be phototoxic. This means that they can cause your skin to discolor or break out in a painful rash after contact with the sun. Some people are very allergic to perfumes and deodorants.

Chew Food for Smooth Neck and Jaw

Dr. J. DeWitt Fox was recently quoted in a newspaper article as suggesting that his patients chew gum. The chewing action, if it is done correctly and the bite is good, will help to firm face, jaw, and neck muscles. In youth, people tend to select hard, crunchy foods, but later in life—perhaps because they do not properly care for their teeth—many people live on a diet of soft foods. The exercise of chewing—really chewing—is good for the jaw and for the glands, and it stimulates the digestive system as well. The following are some good chew-foods that will satisfy a dieter's needs while firming neck and face muscles:

Carrots—big sticks, or a whole firm carrot
The heels of bread—hardened for a few days
Crisp apples—be sure to wash your mouth and brush your teeth after eating
Strips of preserved meat—avoid the ones treated with nitrates if possible
Celery—the stringier the better

If you want to chew gum, select the sugar-free variety; if possible, chew sugar-free bubble gum, which is hard and ungiving. Before you decide to chew gum for exercise, check with your dentist to be sure that you will not be damaging fillings, caps, or crowns.

Partial List Of Sources

Here is a list of sources that will provide products by mail order. I've found these places to be reliable; I hope you like their products.

Cream and Moisturizer, Soap, Elastin, Protein Cream* Catalog:
Jon Suarse Inc.
P.O. Box 634 F.D.R. Station
New York, NY 10022

How to Make Juice Mask:
J.E. Klement
Acme Juicer Co.
1031 Main Avenue
Clifton, NJ 07011

Vitamin and Mineral Catalog:
L & H
1062 Lexington Avenue
New York, NY 10021

Water:
Mountain Valley Water Co.
150 Central Avenue
Hot Springs, Arkansas 71901

Take a picture of your neck when starting my exercises, and again after six months and send them to me. Please send me any of your face-saving tips.

M.J. Saffon
P.O. Box 23 Lenox Hill Station
New York, NY 10021

*Protein Cream that has collagen protein in it.

Index

103